AIDS – Meeting the Challenge

Data, Facts, Background

Sonja Weinreich and Christoph Benn

WCC Publications, Geneva

Original German:

AIDS – Eine Krankheit verändert die Welt: Daten – Fakten – Hintergründe
Frankfurt am Main, Verlag Otto Lembeck, 2003

published with the financial support of:
Brot für die Welt
Deutsches Institut für Ärztliche Mission e.V.
Evangelischer Entwicklungsdient
Evangelisches Missionswerk in Deutschland

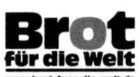 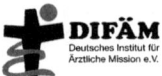 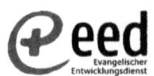

The translation and publication of the English edition were financed by:
Vereinte Evangelische Mission (United Evangelical Mission)

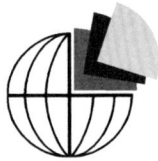

ISBN 2-8254-1351-8

© 2004 World Council of Churches
150 route de Ferney, P.O.Box 2100
1211 Geneva 2, Switzerland
Web site: http://www.wcc-coe.org

Printed in Switzerland

Contents

Preface	ix
Introduction	x

1. Natural history and HIV transmission **1**
    1.1   Natural history 1
    1.2   HIV transmission 2

2. Global, regional and country-specific spread of HIV/AIDS **5**
    2.1   Global 5
    2.2   Africa 8
    2.3   Asia 13
    2.4   Eastern Europe and the Russian Federation 16
    2.5   Latin America and the Caribbean 18
    2.6   High-income countries 19
    2.7   Data collection and sources of information 20

3. Vulnerable population groups **21**
    3.1   Risk and vulnerability 21
    3.2   Migration and mobility 21
    3.3   Wars, conflicts and refugees 22
    3.4   Trafficking in human beings and sex trade 23
    3.5   Commercial sex work 23
    3.6   Injecting drug use 24
    3.7   Men who have sex with men (MSM) 25

4. Gender equity **26**
    4.1   Vulnerability to HIV infection 26
    4.2   Girls and young women 27
    4.3   Gender-based and sexual violence 29
    4.4   Impact of HIV/AIDS on women 29
    4.5   Men 30
            4.5.1 Addressing and involving men 30
            4.5.2 Vulnerability of men and boys 31

5. Children **32**
    5.1   Children living with HIV 32
    5.2   Orphans 32
    5.3   Street children 34
    5.4   Sexual exploitation 34
    5.5   Education on sex and sexuality 34
    5.6   Care and support 35

6. Young people **37**
    6.1   Impact on young people 37
    6.2   Knowledge on sexuality and AIDS 37
    6.3   HIV/AIDS education 37

7. Socio-economic context **40**
    7.1   Poverty, development and socio-economic impact 40
    7.2   Poverty and health 41

7.3	Agricultural sector and food security	42
7.4	Education sector	43
7.5	Health sector	45

8. Stigma and discrimination 46
    8.1   HIV-associated stigma and discrimination 46
    8.2   Denial 47
    8.3   Sexuality and taboo 47
    8.4   Overcoming stigma 47
    8.5   Demystifying HIV/AIDS 48

9. Human rights 50
    9.1   Human rights framework 50
    9.2   International obligations in the human rights context 51
    9.3   Public health and human rights 51

10. People living with HIV/AIDS (PLWHA) 53

11. Prevention 55
    11.1   Significance of prevention 55
    11.2   Effective prevention 55
    11.3   Prevention programmes 58
    11.4   Information, education and communication 59
    11.5   Voluntary Counselling and Testing (VTC) 60
            11.5.1 Preventive effect 60
            11.5.2 VCT programmes 61
            11.5.3 Disclosure of test results 62
            11.5.4 Pre-marital testing 62
    11.6   Condoms 63
            11.6.1 Male condoms 63
            11.6.2 Female condoms 64
            11.6.3 Attitude about condoms 65
    11.7   Male circumcision 66
    11.8   Microbicides 66
    11.9   Prevention and treatment of tuberculosis 67
    11.10 Treatment of sexually transmitted infections (STI) 68
    11.11 Blood transfusions 68
    11.12 Vaccine research 69

12. Mother-to-child HIV transmission (MTCT) 70
    12.1   Risk reduction 71
    12.2   Problems for affected women 71
    12.3   Current recommendations 72

13. Care 74
    13.1   Continuum of care 74
    13.2   Interdependence of prevention and care 74
    13.3   Home base care 75
    13.4   Hospitals and health centres 77
    13.5   Hospices 77
    13.6   Traditional medicine 78

14. Antiretroviral therapy 79
    14.1   Antiretroviral drugs (ARV) 79
    14.2   Access to ARV 80

14.3	Drug prices	82
14.4	Patents	83
14.5	Cost-effectiveness	84
14.6	Ethics	85
14.7	Adherence and treatment literacy	86
14.8	Benefits of increased access to ARV	86

15. HIV/AIDS on the international agenda 88
    15.1   International commitment 88
    15.2   Global Fund to Fight AIDS, Tuberculosis and Malaria 89

16. Advocacy and lobbying 92

17. Culture and tradition 93
    17.1   Biomedical, religious and traditional framework 93
    17.2   Integration of the paradigms 96

18. Churches, theology and HIV/AIDS 98
    18.1   Churches and AIDS 98
    18.2   Activities and initiatives 99
            18.2.1 Ecumenical Advocacy Alliance 99
            18.2.2 Ecumenical HIV Initiative in Africa 99
            18.2.3 South Asia Ecumenical Partnership Programme 99
            18.2.4 Ecumenical Pharmaceutical Network 100
    18.3   Responsibilities, successes and potentials 100
    18.4   Theological aspects 102
            18.4.1 Acceptance and stigma 102
            18.4.2 Sexuality 103
            18.4.3 The church as the body of Christ 104

19. Mainstreaming HIV/AIDS 106
    19.1   What is mainstreaming HIV/AIDS? 106
    19.2   Organizational level 107
    19.3   Programme implementation level 108

20. Literature 110

Preface

> "... for he had healed many, so that all who had diseases pressed upon him to touch him." – *Mark 3:10 (RSV)*

Since the onset of the AIDS pandemic, the churches and agencies of the ecumenical movement have maintained a focus on this global crisis.

From 1986 onwards the WCC has developed recommendations and specific guidelines and resource material on the various facets of HIV/AIDS. In 1996 the WCC Study on AIDS was commissioned by the central committee of the Council – which culminated in the adoption of the statement, "The Impact of HIV/AIDS and Churches' Response" and the publication of *Facing AIDS: The Challenge, the Churches Response*. This policy framework challenged the member churches to face the issue of HIV/AIDS in a forthright and inclusive manner and to initiate definitive action. This was followed by the strengthening of educational processes through theological institutes and lay networks. The launching of the Ecumenical Advocacy Alliance and the Ecumenical HIV/AIDS Initiative for Africa have been significant milestones since then. All these initiatives have been vital to ensure that the churches are focused and on track in the struggle to break the silence and to overcome the disease. The WCC and its membership have developed various resource materials catering to the specific needs of churches in addressing the issue.

AIDS – Meeting the Challenge is an offering to churches and the world – a significant and vital addition to the continuum of knowledge – that will greatly assist churches to be effective and efficient in the struggle to overcome HIV/AIDS. It is a compilation of historical, scientific and statistical material aimed at providing the churches and their partners with a better understanding of the dynamics of HIV/AIDS as well as current information to aid in collaborative efforts at answering the challenge of the disease. The topics include HIV prevention, treatment, counseling, particular concerns of such segments of the population as women and the young, attitudinal changes within churches and society, education, advocacy and the improvement of mechanisms for working together, building on one another's research, experiences and successes. On a practical level this response is deliberately multi-faceted and interactive, encouraging churches and Christian service organizations to build and support coalitions dedicated to overcoming this epidemic.

To be Christ-like we need not only to be sensitive to the needs of our society. We also need to be willing to learn, to be equipped and to act appropriately in mitigating the suffering that is going on. This book will assist us in the mission to continue responding to God's call to engage in ministries of "healing" in the broadest sense, affecting individuals, families, communities and societies.

The German Institute for Medical Missions (DIFAEM) in Tübingen has been crucial in both the development of the Christian Medical Commission in 1968 and the subsequent evolution of the health and healing work at the WCC, including the ecumenical movement's method of addressing the issue of HIV/AIDS. This publication shows their continued capacity to sense the needs of churches worldwide and their commitment and capacity to respond to them. We are grateful to Sonja Weinreich and Christoph Benn for having drawn from a wealth of experiences in the fight against AIDS to write this significant resource book.

Samuel Kobia
General Secretary
World Council of Churches

Introduction

It is universally agreed that HIV/AIDS constitutes one of the most serious threats to human life in our era, and represents one of the greatest problems for the socio-economic development of many countries. All forces must therefore be united to do everything possible to counter this catastrophe.

This booklet seeks to give an overview of the current state of knowledge about HIV/AIDS. A glance at the table of contents suffices to indicate the wide range of problem areas it addresses. HIV/AIDS is a disease which affects almost every aspect of human life. The causes lie in the social, economic and political spheres. Basic medical knowledge is necessary for understanding the disease and the possibilities for treatment. As an illness which is primarily transmitted by sexual contact, a large number of psychological, religious and ethnological aspects need to be taken into consideration. For effective prevention and control, one must draw upon knowledge from educational science, health pedagogy and group dynamics.

It is impossible to present comprehensively all of these aspects and fields of knowledge in a relatively brief document, which can only serve as an introduction. An extensive bibliography invites the reader to review the facts presented and to explore the subject in greater detail. However, virtually no other scientific topic is currently undergoing such rapid change as HIV/AIDS. Even specialists can scarcely keep up with the flood of publications. We have tried to find and present the most up-to-date information. Nevertheless, it is possible that much of this information will be outdated within a short time, or become a focus of disputes in the specialized literature.

The booklet is structured in such a way that it can be used as a reference work: it does not necessarily have to be read in its entirety. Individual sections should also be understandable on their own. For this reason there may be occasional repetitions.

It is the sincere wish of the authors – both of whom have witnessed first-hand and over the course of many years the indescribable human misery caused by HIV/AIDS in Africa – that this booklet will contribute to its more effective control.

Sonja Weinreich
Christoph Benn
Tübingen, Germany

1. Natural history and HIV transmission

1.1 Natural history

- Infections with HIV are caused by two types of virus: HIV-1 and HIV-2. On the molecular level the virus is constantly changing. In order to classify its genetic variability, HIV-1 was divided into several subgroups: M, O and N.

- The M subgroup is further subdivided into 11 subtypes or clades, which appear with regional differences. Subtype B is found more extensively in Europe and America. Subtype C is found in Southern Africa, India and Ethiopia. It is the most widespread subtype and is responsible for 50 per cent of all new infections. The subtypes A, C, D and E are responsible for most of the infections in Africa and Southeast Asia. HIV-2 is found predominantly in Western Africa and, according to the studies conducted thus far, appears to be less aggressive than HIV-1. Double infections do occur.

  > Subtypes or clades of HIV-1 appear with regional differences.

- The incubation period (i.e. the period from infection with the virus until the appearance of disease symptoms) is relatively long. If a person is in otherwise good health, it can take an average of 10 years. There are indications that this phase is somewhat shorter in Africa. That is due inter alia to the frequently encountered malnutrition and reduced access to medical treatment. Among newborns and small children the incubation period can be substantially shorter, because their immune systems are not yet fully mature.

- A few weeks after infection with HIV, some patients develop a flu-like clinical picture, the "acute retroviral syndrome". However, generally, patients do not link this to HIV infection, and it only rarely leads to more extensive diagnostic efforts.

- An HIV infection can be demonstrated through various examination methods:
  - Already after 1–2 weeks the HIV p24 antigen can be detected in the blood. After the formation of the antibodies, the p24 antigen test generally turns negative once again.
  - A specific test (PCR = polymerase chain reaction) is used to detect the virus in the blood, which likewise already reacts 1–2 weeks after the infection.
  - After an average of 6–8 weeks, the organism begins to produce specific antibodies against HIV. Only thereafter can possible antibodies be detected in the blood by anti-HIV tests. The time between the moment of infection and the proof of antibodies is called the window period.

  > After 6–8 weeks, anti-HIV tests can detect antibodies in the blood.

- The antibodies that are produced against the virus are not able to fight off the disease completely, as they can in other viral infections. They can be used, however, to determine if an HIV infection is present.

- The HIV tests normally used check for the presence of antibodies, not the virus itself. If the patient is still in the window period, it can be that an HIV infection is present but the test result is negative.

- After an infection, the HIV test remains positive for life, since the virus no longer disappears from the organism, not even under antiretroviral therapy. In very rare cases, with highly limited immune defences, an HIV test can again turn negative. In such cases the virus is still present, but no more antibodies are being produced.
- In babies born of an HIV-positive mother, up to 18 months after birth the HIV test is always positive, since they have antibodies from the mother which are detected by the test. Only after this period does an HIV test actually make sense, since only then do infants' own antibody production indicate whether they are HIV-positive or HIV-negative.
- HIV rapid tests are less specific than the conventional ELISA tests, but they offer the advantage that the results can be back in just a few minutes, and they can also be performed with limited laboratory equipment. This makes them suitable for use in resource-poor settings.
- AIDS is a syndrome of various symptoms and clinical pictures, caused by the weakening of the immune system as a result of an infection with HIV. It is the last stage of HIV disease, and is characterized by the appearance of a multitude of opportunistic infections, resulting from the breakdown of the immune system. These include pneumonias, skin diseases, diarrhoeal diseases and various forms of neurological infections. Other neurological symptoms include loss of memory and difficulties in walking. In addition, particular forms of tumours, such as Kaposi's sarcoma, develop more frequently than in healthy persons. In Africa, tuberculosis is the most common opportunistic infection. The median survival time after an AIDS-defining complication is 1.3 years, in the absence of antiretroviral therapy.

> AIDS is the last stage of HIV disease, and is characterized by the appearance of opportunistic infections.

- The virus attacks CD4 cells (helper cells) specifically and uses them for its own reproduction. CD4 cells are a subgroup of the white blood cells. The standard value lies between 600–1300 cells/µl of blood. In this process of virus reproduction and subsequent release the CD4 cells are destroyed.
- The number of CD4 cells is a measure for the immunological responsiveness of the organism, for the progress of the HIV infection and for the response to specific therapy with antiretroviral drugs. Generally, the cells decline steadily for around 4–6 years after the infection, until the complete collapse of the immune system. CD4 cell values of <200 cells/µl are "AIDS-defining" and an indication for antiretroviral therapy.

> The number of CD4 cells is a measure of the progress of the HIV infection and of the response to specific therapy with antiretroviral drugs.

- Viral load (quantitative plasma HIV RNA) measures the amount of virus in the blood. It is used for the diagnosis of acute HIV infection, for predicting probability of transmission, predicting the rate of progression in chronically infected patients, and for therapeutic monitoring.

1.2 HIV TRANSMISSION

- All forms of HIV are transmitted via four different infection routes:
  - Sexual intercourse (vaginal, anal, oral).
  - Blood and blood products.
  - Needles and other skin-piercing instruments.

- Mother-to-child transmission from an HIV-infected woman during pregnancy, during childbirth or through breast milk (perinatal transmission).
- The probabilities for an HIV transmission vary greatly depending on the transmission route.
  - In general, the risk of transmission of HIV by an infected to an uninfected partner through sexual intercourse for a one-time sexual contact lies substantially lower than is widely assumed, at an average of 0.01 per cent (Gray et al. 2001). This risk increases with a high virus concentration in the blood (e.g. with advanced HIV disease) and in the presence of sexually transmitted infections, yet remains below 1 per cent.
  - It is generally assumed that there is a higher risk for the infection route from male to female than vice versa. A study from Uganda (Gray et al. 2001) could not confirm this trend, however. Nevertheless, the risk of HIV infection is higher for girls, since their genital organs are not yet mature, and is higher for females if sex takes place violently.
  - Studies have shown that the risk after an injury with a needle which was in contact with infected blood amounts to 0.3 per cent (Henderson et al. 1990). Thus, for surgeons in Zambia, the risk of infecting themselves with HIV is 15 times higher than for colleagues in Europe (Consten et al. 1995).
  - Post-exposure prophylaxis is available to reduce the likelihood of an infection after exposure to a contaminated instrument, and increasingly also to survivors of sexual violence.
  - A blood transfusion with infected blood has the highest transmission probability (>90%), since in this case large quantities of infected blood enter directly into the recipient's bloodstream.
  - With mother-to-child transmission of HIV, the probability depends on several factors, and varies between <2% in the industrialized countries and >30% in developing countries.
- Almost 87 per cent of all HIV infections in Africa are transmitted through heterosexual intercourse, with lower proportions due to blood transfusions (2 per cent), intravenous drug use (1 per cent) and mother-to-child (10 per cent).
- WHO suspects that up to 5 per cent of all HIV infections might be transmitted through unsterile needles and other equipment. It has been argued that the proportion of infections through contaminated blood products (in the hospital, with private doctors and traditional healers) could be substantially higher (Gisselquist et al. 2003). More thorough studies need to be done on this.
- Heterosexual transmission is a growing route in Western countries, as well as in Asia, Latin America and Northern Africa/Middle East. The following graphs show estimates of the proportions of transmission routes in Africa and the industrialized countries (in percentage terms) (according to the Global AIDS Surveillance 2001):

> The risk of HIV transmission resulting from a one-time sexual contact is 0.01 per cent. 87 per cent of all HIV infections in Africa are transmitted through heterosexual intercourse. This is also an increasing transmission route in the industrialized countries.

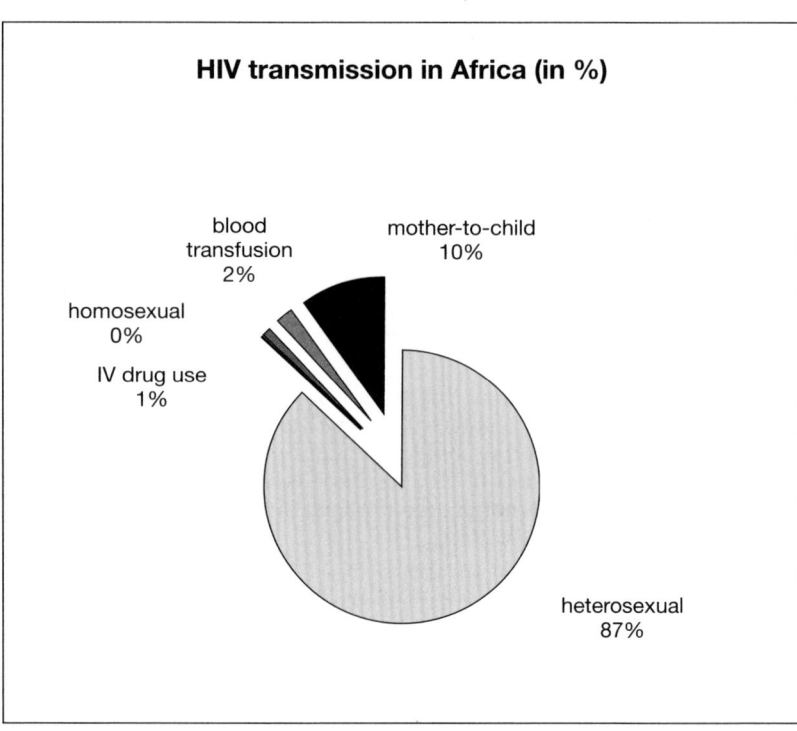
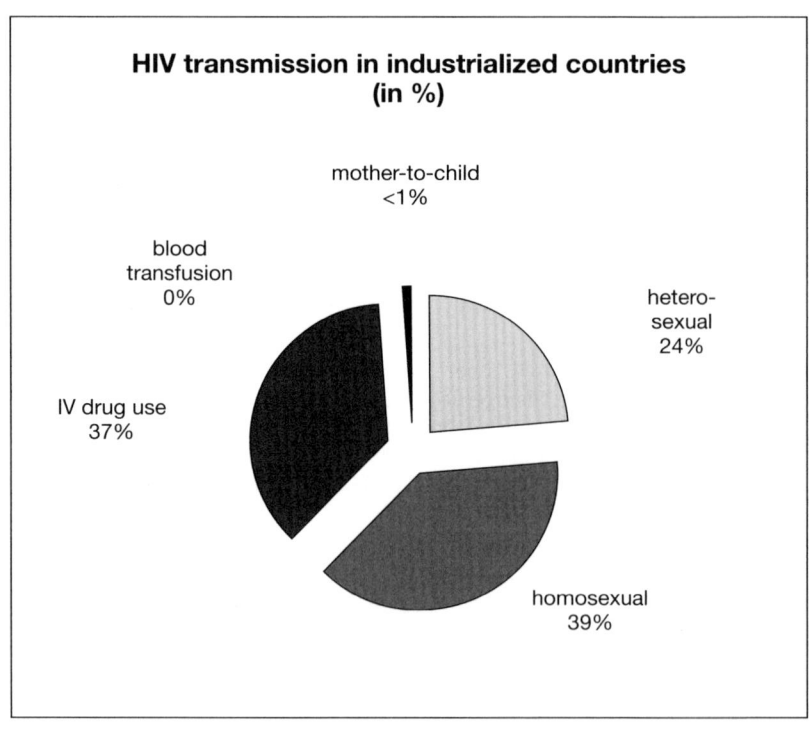

2. Global, regional and country-specific spread of HIV/AIDS

2.1 GLOBAL

- UNAIDS, the Joint United Nations Programme on AIDS, together with WHO, issues epidemiological reports on a regular basis. The "Report on the global HIV/AIDS epidemic 2002" from July 2002 gave HIV data for regions and individual countries for 2001 (UNAIDS 2002), and the "AIDS epidemic update" from November 2003 contains global and regional data for 2003 (UNAIDS 2003). Further country-specific data for 2003 was published in mid-2004.
- Since the appearance of the first HIV cases in 1981, more than 60 million people have been infected with the virus, around 20 million of whom have died.
- In the year 2003, throughout the world around 40 million people were living with HIV; 5 million people were newly infected; 3 million died of AIDS.
- More than 90 per cent of all HIV infected persons live in developing countries.
- It has become evident that the HIV/AIDS pandemic (epidemic on a world scale) is only in the initial stages, and the course which it will take over the long term is not yet sufficiently clear. Although the epidemic has developed explosively thus far, its dynamic must be considered over a time scale of decades.
- The world is facing a multitude of AIDS epidemics, which differ in their time sequences, extent and the affected populations. In many countries the epidemic is still "low" or "concentrated" and limited to groups with especially high risk, including homosexuals, drug users and commercial sex workers.
- An HIV epidemic is "concentrated" when less than 1 per cent of the general population, but more than 5 per cent of the "high-risk groups", are infected. When more than 1 per cent of the general population is infected, the epidemic tends to spread rapidly. Such generalized epidemics are found in Africa, parts of Asia, Central America and the Caribbean (UNICEF/UNAIDS/WHO 2002).

> In the year 2003, 40 million people around the world were living with HIV; 5 million were newly infected with HIV, which amounts to 13,700 per day; 3 million died of AIDS – 8,500 per day.

- The following table presents global data for 2003 for adults and children (UNAIDS 2003):

Region	HIV infections	Prevalence	AIDS deaths	New infections
Global	40 million (34–46 million)	1.1% (0.9–1.3%)	3 million (2.5–3.3 million)	5 million (4.2–5.8 million)
Sub-Saharan Africa	25.0–28.2 million	7.5–8.5%	2.2–2.4 million	3.0–3.4 million
Northern Africa & Middle East	470 000–730 000	0.2–0.4%	35,000–50,000	43,000–67,000
South Asia & Southeast Asia	4.6–8.2 million	0.4–0.8 %	330,000–590,000	610,000–1 million
East Asia & Pacific	700,000–1.3 million	0.1%	32,000–58,000	150,000–270,000
Latin America	1.3–1.9 million	0.5–0.7%	49,000–70,000	120,000–180,000
Caribbean	350,000–590,000	1.9–3.1%	30,000–50,000	45,000–80,000
Eastern Europe & Central Asia	1.2–11.8 million	0.5–0.9%	23,000–37,000	180,000–280,000
Western Europe	520,000–680,000	0.3%	2,600–3,400	30,000–40,000
North America	790,000–1.2 million	0.5–0.7%	12,000–18,000	36,000–54,000
Australia	12,000–18,000	0.1%	<100	700–1,000

- The proportion of women among HIV-infected persons worldwide has grown continuously over the years, with rising absolute figures. In the year 2002 one-half of all HIV-infected adults were women. One essential reason for this is that, although women are more vulnerable to HIV infection, it is largely men who determine sexual behaviour.
- In regions where HIV transmission was primarily determined by heterosexual contacts, the proportion of women was higher from the start. Here too, however, one finds a more-than-proportional increase in the women's share, as in Africa. Where HIV is primarily transmitted among drug users, more men were initially affected. But here HIV is spreading to female drug users and to female sexual partners.

> The proportion of women among HIV-infected persons worldwide has grown continuously over the years.

- The following table gives the corresponding values (sources: UNAIDS 1998, 2000, 2002):

	HIV+ve adults & children			% women among HIV +ve adults		
Region	*1997*	*2000*	*2002*	*1997*	*2000*	*2002*
Sub-Saharan Africa	20.8 m	25.3 m	29.4 m	50	55	58
South Asia & Southeast Asia	6 m	5.8 m	6 m	25	35	36
Western Europe & USA	1.4 m	1.4 m	1.4 m	20	20–25	20–25
Eastern Europe	150,000	700,000	1 m	25	25	27
Total	**30.6 m**	**36.1 m**	**40 m**	**41**	**47**	**50**

- A report published in September 2002 by the National Intelligence Council of the US, which also incorporated data from unofficial sources and NGOs, sees five countries around the world which in the coming decade will be most strongly affected by HIV/AIDS: Ethiopia, Nigeria, India, China and Russia. These countries together constitute 40 per cent of the world's population (NIC 2002).
- AIDS-related deaths are increasing globally (UNAIDS 2003):

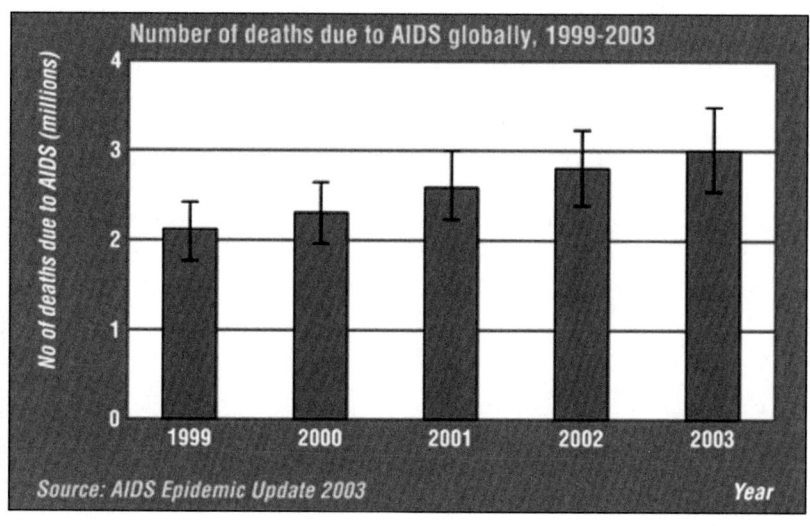

2.2 Africa

> In 2003 in sub-Saharan Africa 26.6 million people were infected with HIV, 2.3 million died of AIDS and 3.2 million were newly infected.

- Worldwide, the region most severely affected is sub-Saharan Africa, where more than two-thirds (26.6 million) of all HIV-infected people live. In the year 2003 in Africa alone 2.3 million people died of AIDS (i.e. more than 6,500 people every day) and 3.2 million people were newly infected with HIV.
- Thus, this region – with 10 per cent of the world's population – has 70 per cent of all HIV-infected persons and 77 per cent of all AIDS-related deaths.
- HIV/AIDS is the most frequent cause of death in sub-Saharan Africa.

> In several countries, the lifetime risk of becoming infected with HIV is over 60 per cent.

- The life expectancy in sub-Saharan Africa is 47 years; without AIDS, it would be 62. However, the risk (related to the full lifetime) of being infected with HIV is even higher than the data on prevalence would lead one to believe. In Botswana, South Africa and Zimbabwe an estimated 60 per cent of the young men who today are 15 years old will be infected with HIV during the course of their lifetimes, if prevention efforts do not succeed.
- Data for South Africa show that in the 1990s there was a steady increase in the death rates among adults, and that in the year 2000 approximately 40 per cent of deaths among adults were conditioned in some way by HIV/AIDS (South African Medical Research Council 2001).
- The government of Botswana estimates that, without adequate treatment, one-third of the population will die of AIDS during the course of the next 10 years. The most pessimistic estimates proceed on the assumption that, by the year 2010, life expectancy will have decreased to 29 years. The current statistics indicate that one-half of all households in Botswana have an HIV-positive family member. It is expected that in the future, for every breadwinner, there will be four additional dependent persons, and that by the year 2010 20 per cent of all children will be orphans (Botswana 2000).

> The epidemic has no natural limit above which the infections will no longer increase.

- While it was first assumed that the epidemic would reach a "natural limit," we are now seeing that this is not the case. For example, in Botswana the HIV prevalence among pregnant women in urban areas in 1997 was 38.5 per cent and by 2001 it had risen to 44 per cent.
- 12 African countries have infection rates of more than 10 per cent of the adult population; 7 of these, most in Southern Africa, are over 20 per cent.

- The following table shows the number of HIV-infected adults and children and the corresponding prevalences in several African countries for the year 2001 (source: UNAIDS 2002):

Country	HIV infections	Prevalence (%)
Angola	350,000	5.0
Benin	120,000	3.6
Botswana	330,000	38.8
Burkina Faso	440,000	6.5
Burundi	390,000	8.3
Cameroon	920,000	11.8
Central African Republic	250,000	12.9
Congo	110,000	7.2
Congo (Dem. Rep.)	1,300,000	4.9
Côte d'Ivoire	770,000	9.7
Eritrea	55,000	2.8
Ethiopia	2,100,000	6.4
Ghana	360,000	3.0
Kenya	2,000,000	15.0
Lesotho	360,000	31.0
Malawi	850,000	15.0
Mozambique	1,100,000	13.0
Namibia	230,000	22.5
Nigeria	3,500,000	5.8
Rwanda	500,000	8.9
Senegal	27,000	0.5
Sierra Leone	170,000	7.0
South Africa	5,000,000	20.1
Swaziland	170,000	33.4
Tanzania	1,500,000	7.8
Uganda	600,000	5.0
Zambia	1,200,000	21.5
Zimbabwe	2,300,000	33.7

- In some age groups the prevalence is even higher than the average figures suggest. Generally, it is highest among women in the age groups 20–29 years, and among men between 30–39 years.
- The following graph shows HIV prevalence among pregnant women in Namibia by age groups, from 1994 to 2000 (source: Erskine 2001):

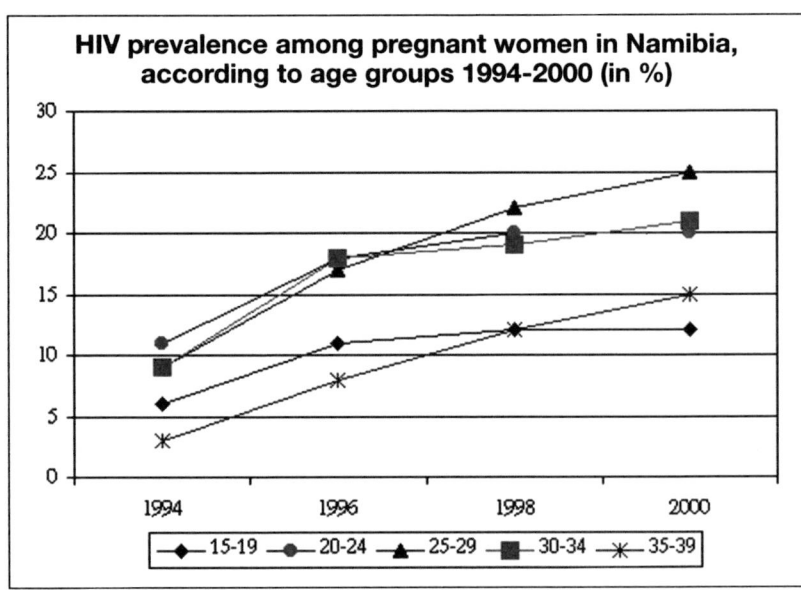

- HIV prevalences often show significant differences within the regions, and are generally higher in urban than in rural areas. However, in many countries the rural rates are approaching the urban rates.

- The following graph shows HIV prevalences in South Africa 1992–2000 (source: South Africa 2000):

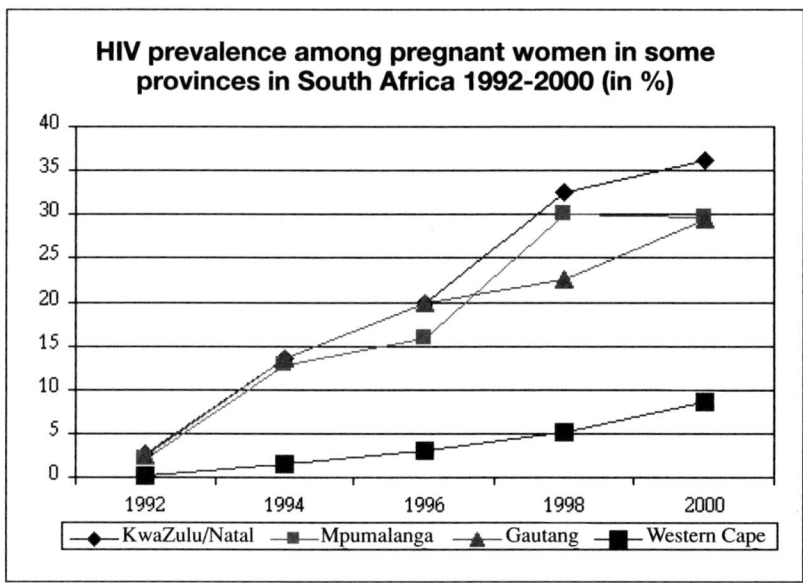

- The report of the South African government for the year 2001 gives prevalence by age groups for pregnant women, which is interpreted as a decline in the incidence among young people (South Africa 2002). However, it remains to be seen whether this trend will continue.
- The South African Human and Social Research Council (2002) investigated HIV prevalence through representative samples from the overall population. It found a surprisingly high prevalence among 2–14 year olds, at 5.6 per cent. Further research is required in this context.
- In Western and Central Africa there are indications of a recent rapid spread of HIV. Eight countries in this region have an HIV prevalence >5%.
- In Cameroon the prevalence has risen sharply in recent years. In urban areas it amounted to 2 per cent in 1998, 4.7 per cent in 1996 and 11.8 per cent in 2001. This could be the beginning of a further steep increase, especially since the highest prevalence is found among younger women, and the prevalence in urban and rural areas is at virtually the same level.

> Cameroon has a sharply rising HIV epidemic: the prevalence rose from 4.7 per cent in 1996 to 11.8 per cent in 2001.

- Nigeria is showing a slowly rising prevalence: from 1.9 per cent in 1993 to 5.8 per cent in 2001. Some federal states in Nigeria, however, have substantially higher prevalences, and a total of more than 3 million people in Nigeria are living with HIV.
- In sub-Saharan Africa approximately twice as many young women as men are infected: in 2001, 6–11 per cent of the women between 15 and 24 years were infected with HIV, compared with 3–6 per cent of the men in this age group (see chapter 4 on gender equity).

> In sub-Saharan Africa twice as many women are infected as men in the age group of 15–24 year olds.

- The majority of HIV-infected persons in Africa lack adequate medical care for treatment of opportunistic infections, and less than 1 per cent have access to life-prolonging antiretroviral drugs.
- A mature HIV epidemic is only now establishing itself in many countries, since many people who in recent years have been infected with HIV are falling sick and dying. Without adequate care and treatment, deaths will increase in the coming years and their greatest number will only be reached towards the end of the decade. This means that the most ominous consequences of the epidemic will only become noticeable in the course of this decade and after.
- However, there are also indications that in several of the most affected countries (e.g. Zambia and Uganda) HIV prevention is having an impact.
- In Zambia in recent years, the number of HIV infections among 15–19 year olds has declined, particularly among the girls in this age group. This is presumably due to changes in sexual behaviour, since there are indications of an increased use of condoms, a decline in the number of sexual partners and an increase in the age when women have their first child (Fylkesnes et al. 2001). Given the lack of political commitment to combating AIDS, the vigorous participation of community organizations and churches in HIV prevention has contributed to the successes.
- In Uganda, HIV prevalence fell from 14 per cent in the earlier 1990s to 5 per cent in the year 2001. In the urban areas, the rates of new infections have fallen by 50 per cent. The decline was sharpest in the age group of 15–19 year olds. Among other things, this decline is due to the fact that the commencement of sexual activity among young people has been delayed by an average of 2 years, the number of sexual partners declined and the reported use of condoms increased. Thus, prevention campaigns are having an effect.
- Uganda is seen as demonstrating the fact that even a mature HIV epidemic can be brought under control. The national reaction to AIDS was collective and encompassed all levels of the government, NGOs, religious groups, communities and international sponsors. Successes are not based on a single prevention strategy; rather, strategies were applied in a continuum: the establishment of AIDS control programmes in ministries, the formulation of a national AIDS policy, capacity building in institutions and organizations, inclusion of civil society (including faith-based organizations), education campaigns, reduction of stigmatization, provision of condoms, screening of blood transfusions, access to VCT, care for orphans, treatment of opportunistic infections and sexually transmitted infections.
- However, the impact of AIDS in Uganda still entails high social and economic costs. For example, incomes and food security for a large part of the population are not ensured, and the orphan crisis will generate serious problems for many years to come (Asiimwe-Akiror et al. 1997; Okware et al. 2001; UNAIDS 2002).

Best Practice

TASO

The AIDS Support Organization (TASO) was founded in 1987 in Kampala as an NGO by several people who were personally affected by HIV/AIDS. Since then, six further centres have been added in various places in Uganda. Since its foundation TASO has provided medical, material and social care to more than 60,000 HIV-infected people and their families, and through AIDS education and awareness raising reaches 100,000 people per year. In addition, the organization provides counselling for individuals, families and communities and promotes capacity building for fighting AIDS within the communities. Training of HIV counsellors is conducted throughout Uganda, as well as for other countries. TASO receives the greatest share of its financial support through European governmental and North American development aid organizations. TASO has demonstrated that participation of the communities, together with international expertise and resources, are of central importance for combating the HIV epidemic (TASO 2001).

> Uganda is seen as demonstrating the fact that even a mature HIV epidemic can be brought under control. A collective national response to the epidemic also included NGOs and faith-based organizations.

- Senegal undertook extensive prevention efforts at an early stage of the epidemic, and it still has a relatively low HIV prevalence of 0.5 per cent. The inclusion of faith-based organizations played an important role in the success (UNAIDS 2002).

> Senegal has a low prevalence of 0.5 per cent after early prevention.

2.3 ASIA

- In 2003 an estimated 7.4 million people were living with HIV in Asia and the Pacific region. Over 1 million were newly infected with HIV during the course of the year 2003.

> In 2003, 7.4 million people were living with HIV in Asia.

- According to projections, of the 45 million infections expected by the year 2010, 40 per cent will take place in Asia, while currently 20 per cent of the new infections occur there. The following graph shows the increase in HIV infections from 1996 to 2001 (source: UNAIDS/WHO):

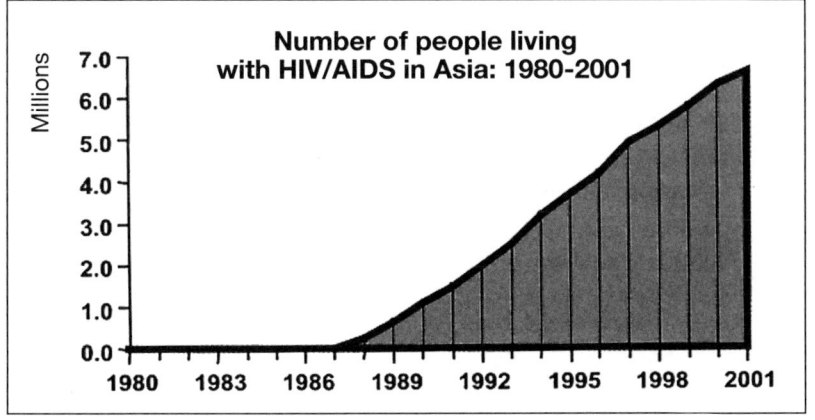

Source: UNAIDS/WHO, 2002

- In Asia, the primary transmission routes for HIV are heterosexual intercourse, needle sharing among drug users, and men who have sex with men. Poverty, an increasing sex trade, drug use, a high rate of sexually transmitted infections and large population movements contribute to increased vulnerability to HIV infection in this region.

> Generalized HIV epidemics are developing in Indonesia, Nepal, India, China and Vietnam.

- Three countries – Cambodia, Myanmar and Thailand – have national prevalence rates of more than 1 per cent. However, initially concentrated epidemics among drug users and commercial sex workers (CSWs) are spreading into the general population in Indonesia, Nepal, India, China and Vietnam, following the pattern in Cambodia and Thailand several years ago (MAP 2001, UNAIDS 2003).

- Relatively low national HIV prevalences can conceal localized HIV epidemics and the risk that the epidemic is spreading.

  - In most countries, HIV epidemics are concentrated in certain population groups. In Myanmar, for example, the HIV rates among CSWs and drug users run as high as 60 per cent, although the national average in the general population is only 2 per cent.

> In 2001 the prevalence in India was 0.8 per cent. However, in several areas the epidemic is spreading from the high-risk groups into the general population.

  - In India approximately 3.9 million people are living with HIV/AIDS. India is thus the country with the greatest HIV epidemic in Asia and has, after South Africa, worldwide the highest number of HIV-positive people. In 2001 the national HIV prevalence, at 0.8 per cent, was relatively low. However, in Andra Pradesh, Karnataka, Maharashtra, Manipur, Nagaland and Tamil Nadu >1% of pregnant women are HIV-positive. This means that in several areas the epidemic is spreading into the general population.

  - Through the type of spread of HIV (i.e. individual-to-individual through sex and shared use of injection equipment among drug users), epidemics first begin in geographically limited areas and then spread into the rest of the population. Drug users frequently have commercial sex or sex with other partners who are not using drugs. Many CSWs also inject illicit drugs. Condom use is generally low among all these groups.

  - National HIV data are not very meaningful in countries like China and India, which are so populous that some of their federal states have more inhabitants than do some other countries.

  - In several cases, poor data collection puts the reliability of the data into question.

- In order to make forecasts about the future course of the HIV/AIDS epidemic in Asia, local data should be used in addition to national data, and one should study how the epidemic has developed in other regions (e.g. in Africa).

- Despite the difficulty of making precise forecasts, it is clear that there is no (naturally occurring) upper limit for the HIV prevalence. In Thailand and Cambodia, for example, even after years of the HIV epidemic, HIV prevalence lies below 2 per cent. This is probably due more to the effectiveness of implemented prevention programmes than to a naturally occurring limitation of the epidemic.

- For Cambodia, there are indications that prevention among sex workers has caused condom use to increase and the number of HIV infections in this group to fall from 42 per cent in 1998 to 29 per cent in 2002.
- In 2001 the HIV prevalence in Thailand was 1.8 per cent. Thailand implemented a successful "100% condom strategy" which reduced the annual number of new infections from 140,000 in 1990 to 30,000 in 2000. This strategy included a package of measures and activities: discussion of sexual behaviour on a national scale, structural solutions such as regulation of the sex industry, intensive education, peer interventions among CSWs and activities targeting their clients. Thanks to these interventions, the percentage of men visiting CSWs fell by one-half, and condom use in these sexual contacts rose from 10 per cent to 90 per cent (Kilmarx et al. 2000).

  > In 2001 the prevalence in Thailand was 1.8 per cent. Thailand has for many years conducted successful prevention, with the focus on condom use among CSWs and further supporting measures.

- Infection rates can rise quickly, even after they have remained at a low level for years. Low HIV infection rates at the present time are no guarantee for low infection rates in the future.
- In 2001 Nepal had an HIV prevalence of 0.5 per cent. However, migration and drug use are important factors for HIV dissemination. In the early 1990s in Katmandu there were a large number of drug users, yet virtually no HIV infections. During the following years, however, the infection exploded among drug users, and in 1997 the HIV prevalence in this group reached 50 per cent.
- Because of the danger of localized HIV epidemics turning into large, generalized epidemics, HIV prevention in Asia has decisive significance. In prevention, the specific vulnerable groups (CSWs, drug users, etc.) must be addressed. However, the general population must also be targeted by prevention interventions.
- The example of Thailand makes this necessity clear: thanks to prevention programmes, HIV transmission from CSWs to their clients dropped from 77 per cent in 1990 to 12 per cent in 2000. However, HIV transmission from male clients to their wives, who were not regarded as a target group in the HIV prevention programme, rose from 5 per cent to 18 per cent. While in the 1990s the greatest share of HIV transmissions came through commercial sex, half of all new infections are now occurring among the female partners of men who were infected some years earlier.

  > In Asia prevention has decisive significance. One must reach not only the high-risk groups, but also the general population.

- In large parts of Asia, prevention programmes are not adequately funded. Projects are often implemented only on a small scale, and are scattered across the states. Moreover, stigmatization and criminalization of minorities with great vulnerability to HIV infection (prostitution, drug use, homosexuality) represent serious obstacles for HIV prevention.
- In 2001 China's national HIV prevalence was 0.1 per cent. Reported HIV infections rose by 67 per cent in the first six months of 2001. The official number for 2002 is given as 1 million infected persons. Since monitoring is limited almost exclusively to relatively small high-risk groups, this number presumably underestimates the actual situation. International groups work on the assumption that the number of HIV-infected persons is closer to 1.5 million and that if the epidemic continues to grow at the present rate, this could increase to 20 million by the year 2010. HIV

  > In several provinces in China there are epidemics among drug users which are spreading into the general population.

epidemics exist in at least nine provinces among drug users, whereby in Yunan, for example, the HIV prevalence among drug users is >70%. A further nine provinces are on the threshold of similar epidemics. In Henan province, several tens of thousands of impoverished village inhabitants are HIV-infected. In the 1990s they sold their blood to commercial firms which did not strictly comply with the safety rules for blood transfusions. It is estimated that up to 1 million people may have been infected with HIV in this way (Editorial 2001a). There are fears that similar epidemics exist in other provinces. The opening up of society is bringing with it an increase in prostitution and migration, and a change in the sexual values of young people, which entail a heightened risk of HIV infection: the HIV prevalence among CSWs and patients with sexually transmitted diseases has risen rapidly.

In Indonesia there has been a rapid increase in HIV infections among CSWs, drug users and blood donors.

– In 2001 Indonesia had an HIV prevalence of 0.05 per cent nationwide. The use of illicit drugs was a virtually unknown phenomenon until recently. However, a sharp increase in the number of drug users has been registered, and the number of HIV-positive people in this group has grown rapidly, from 15 per cent in 1999 to 40 per cent in 2000. Moreover, the number of HIV-positive blood donors has also risen, from 0.02 per cent to almost 0.2 per cent. Even if the absolute figures are not dramatic, this sudden tenfold increase is nevertheless alarming. It can be taken as a sign that the epidemic is spreading from these vulnerable groups into the rest of the population (MAP 2001, UNAIDS 2002).

2.4 EASTERN EUROPE AND THE RUSSIAN FEDERATION

Eastern Europe and the Russian Federation have the world's highest growth rates for HIV infections. The number of infected persons is estimated at 1.5 million. The increase is above all conditioned by an epidemic among drug users, which then spreads outward.

– For years, the states of Eastern Europe and the Russian Federation have had the world's highest HIV growth rates. New estimates put the number of HIV-infected persons (including Central Asia) at 1.5 million in the year 2003, of whom some 230,000 were newly infected (UNAIDS 2003).

– In Eastern Europe and the Russian Federation the main transmission route for HIV is needle sharing (around 82 per cent of all HIV infections) and unprotected sexual intercourse among injecting drug users and their partners.

– Illicit drug use especially involves young people in the age group between 15 and 24. In the last 5 years, injecting drug use among young people in the Russian Federation has trebled. The official number of users of various drugs is estimated for 2002 at 2.5–3 million, which is extremely high compared to the total population. The number of injecting heroin users is estimated to be around 1.5 million (United Nations Office for Drug Control 2002). Approximately 1 per cent of the populations of the Eastern European countries use injection drugs.

– Most drug users are men; however, the number of female drug users is probably higher than assumed, since they are still less often registered. Many of them are also engaged in commercial sex.

– The registered HIV cases probably underestimate the actual number of people living with HIV. Sentinel surveillance and counselling and testing centres are inadequate: most HIV tests are performed as part of a

- routine screening when people come into contact with the criminal prosecution authorities or use health facilities.
- The following graph shows the cumulative HIV infections of 1993–2001 (source: UNAIDS):

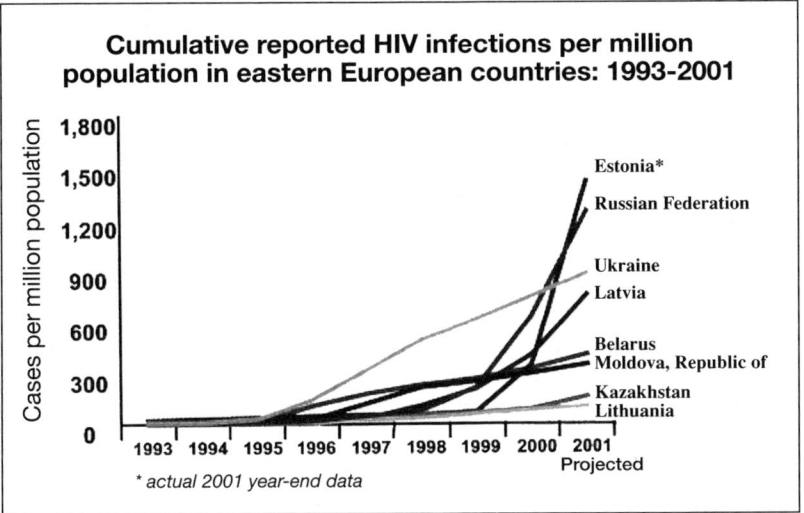

Source: National AIDS Programmes (2001) HIV/AIDS surveillance in Europe. Mid-year report. Data compiled by the European Centre for the Epidemiological Monitoring of AIDS

- The number of officially registered HIV infections in the Russian Federation amounted to more than 230,000, but it is estimated that it is 1 million people in 2003. The infection rate in the adult population is given as 0.9 per cent. The greatest cause for concern, however, is the rate of increase, because since 1998 the number of HIV infections has virtually doubled every year.

> In Russia, the HIV infection rate has doubled annually since 1998.

- The relatively high number of young people in overcrowded prisons where drugs are readily available, but no information about HIV is provided, and where there is no access to clean needles and condoms, also constitutes a breeding ground for the rapid spread of HIV.
- With 1 per cent, Ukraine has the highest HIV prevalence in Eastern Europe, whereby the number of unreported cases could in fact be as much as 10 times higher. While injecting drug use is responsible for around 75 per cent of the infections, the proportion of sexually transmitted HIV infections is increasing.
- Heterosexual intercourse is becoming an increasingly important transmission route. In Kaliningrad 40 per cent of infections are through sexual intercourse, and this trend can be observed in all countries of the region. An important sign is the dramatic increase in other sexually transmitted infections.
- An important transmission route is sexual intercourse among homosexual men, although there are no official statistics on this. Studies have identified high-risk behaviour and a very low awareness about prevention measures. Also unknown is what role is played by transmission via transfusion.

> The epidemic is not only a humanitarian catastrophe, but will also have significant economic effects in Eastern Europe.

- The epidemic is also spreading in Kazakhstan, Azerbaijan, Georgia, Kyrgyzstan, Tajikistan and Uzbekistan.
- It is now becoming clear that the HIV/AIDS epidemic not only represents a humanitarian catastrophe, but will also have significant economic consequences. In a report of the Moscow regional office of the World Bank, a scientific model calculation was used to assess and quantify the overall economic consequences resulting from HIV/AIDS (Ruhl et al. 2002). The economists simulated an optimistic and a pessimistic scenario, according to which without prevention measures the number of HIV-infected persons by the end of 2010 could rise to 2.5 million people, and by 2020 to anywhere between 5.4 and 14.5 million. That would be 4–12 per cent of the present-day population. Under these assumptions, the gross domestic product in the year 2020 would be as much as 10.5 per cent lower than would be the case without AIDS.
- This model calculation should make clear how urgent it is to introduce effective countermeasures. Only by offering prevention and treatment will one succeed in stopping a development which has already occurred in other regions of the world and led to devastating consequences. At the moment the epidemic is still in a relatively early stage, so the implementation of strong prevention measures offers a realistic hope of containing the epidemic.

> Massive prevention efforts are necessary to stop the further spread of the epidemic in Eastern Europe and the Russian Federation.

- Interventions must be targeted at reducing the infection risk of young people in sexual behaviour and in injecting drug use. Above all, harm-reduction programmes have demonstrated their effectiveness, but they are underused.
- Furthermore, one must address the socio-economic factors which encourage the spread of HIV: mass unemployment, change of social and cultural standards and the disintegration of the public healthcare system.

2.5 Latin America and the Caribbean

> After Africa, the Caribbean is the world region which is hardest hit by HIV/AIDS.

- In 2003 more than 2 million people were living with HIV in Latin America and the Caribbean. The Caribbean is – after Africa – the world region most severely affected by HIV/AIDS. Haiti (6 per cent) and the Bahamas (3.5 per cent) have the highest HIV prevalences.
- HIV transmission in these regions takes place predominantly heterosexually, and is propelled by unprotected sexual intercourse and frequent partner change among young people. Social factors which promote the spread of HIV include poor socio-economic conditions and a high population mobility, including tourism.
- Another important transmission route is homosexual contact. In Mexico, the HIV prevalence among men who have sex with men is 14 per cent. Transmission routes can also differ within a country: in the highlands of Colombia HIV is generally transmitted through sexual intercourse between men, and on the coast through heterosexual intercourse.
- A study in seven countries in Central America found HIV prevalences among homosexuals between 8 and 18 per cent. Such men frequently also have sex with women. Thus, prevention programmes cannot concentrate solely on "homosexual behaviour".

- Of growing significance for the spread of HIV is the shared use of injection equipment among drug users: above all in Argentina, Brazil, Chile, Uruguay, Paraguay, Mexico, the Bermudas and Puerto Rico.
- Some countries have government programmes for antiretroviral drugs, although these programmes differ in their nature and scope. The countries which are furthest along in creating access to ARV drugs are Brazil, Argentina and Uruguay. Brazil is also registering a substantial decline in HIV prevalence among intravenous drug users in the major cities, thanks to the successful implementation of prevention and harm-reduction programmes which make safe injection techniques possible (UNAIDS 2001a, 2001b).

2.6 HIGH-INCOME COUNTRIES

- In Western Europe, the USA and Canada, 1.6 million people were living with the virus, and 80,000 were newly infected in 2003. The HIV prevalence in Western Europe was 0.3 per cent and in the US 0.6 per cent (UNAIDS 2002, 2003).

> In 2003, 1.6 million people were living with HIV in the high-income countries.

- Around 500,000 people received ARV treatment in the year 2001. Since the introduction of these combination therapies in 1996, AIDS death rates have fallen by up to 70 per cent. The longer life expectancy has led to a steady increase in the number of HIV-infected persons, while new infection rates have remained virtually constant – however, with a trend to rise over the recent past.
- Diminishing awareness among the public about the risk of HIV infection, plus discontinued prevention programmes, could lead to an expanding epidemic.
- An increase in unprotected intercourse among men who have sex with men entails a risk of higher HIV transmission rates: in San Francisco, the prevalence among homosexuals who also inject drugs rose from 2 per cent in 1997 to 4.6 per cent in 2000.
- In the industrialized countries, the HIV epidemic is moving from certain vulnerable groups (men who have sex with men and drug users) to poorer and marginalized population groups, such as ethnic minorities and immigrants from countries with higher prevalence.
- Also, a greater proportion of the new infections takes place through heterosexual intercourse. In the US, 56 per cent of newly infected persons among 13–19 year olds were female, a disproportionately high share among them female Afro-Americans (UNAIDS 2002).
- In the industrialized countries, mother-to-child transmission represents a tiny fraction of all HIV transmissions because specific measures to reduce the transmission risk are implemented, such as Caesarean sections, specific antiretroviral drugs, and alternatives to breast feeding.

2.7 DATA COLLECTION AND SOURCES OF INFORMATION

Prevalence is the number of existing cases of a disease; *incidence* is the number of newly appearing cases, each related to a specific population.

- The global collection and surveillance of data on HIV/AIDS is a joint undertaking of UNAIDS and WHO, in cooperation with national data collection systems and other organizations. The objective is to gather data which contribute to an understanding of the current situation and trends and which will facilitate assessment of the risk and vulnerability of populations.
- The data give figures and estimates for HIV prevalence and incidence. The prevalence is the number of existing cases at a given point in time related to a population, while incidence is the number of newly occurring cases within a specific period of time related to a population.

Data from antenatal clinics are used as approximate values for the prevalence within the general population. These are brought together with data from representative samples of communities.

- The concept of "adult population" in the data collections is defined as people between 15 and 49 years of age. Data from antenatal clinics are often drawn upon as approximate values for the prevalence within the general population. HIV tests are conducted anonymously for this purpose. Limitations must be considered: only data on the prevalence and incidence among women are gathered, and the data thus acquired tend to under-represent the HIV prevalence within the overall population.
- Studies are also conducted in individual communities on a representative sample of the population, in order to obtain more precise estimates. These data are then compared and brought together in order to obtain more accurate estimates of HIV prevalence within the general population.
- All data are estimates and not precise counts of infections. The methodology used has been substantially improved over the years. It can often provide a good indication of the scope of the epidemic in a country. In many countries, however, data collection is not very accurate.
- When very many deaths occur from AIDS – as is the case in severely affected countries – the prevalence can remain the same despite a high number of newly infected cases. Thus, a deceptive image of a stable epidemiological situation can be generated, since the number of HIV-related deaths offsets the number of new cases.
- Many countries lack reliable statistics on AIDS mortality. It is thus highly probable that many AIDS deaths are not registered as such. For this reason, statistics on AIDS deaths must be evaluated very cautiously.
- UNAIDS publishes updates on global and country-specific epidemiology, collections of Best Practices and so on. The documents can be ordered from UNAIDS in Geneva. Most publications are also available via the UNAIDS website at www.unaids.org. WHO publications can be obtained at www.who.int.

3. Vulnerable population groups

3.1 RISK AND VULNERABILITY

- In the fight against AIDS, the focus has often been on interventions targeted at "risk groups" (e.g. CSWs). However, such interventions have the disadvantage that they might lead to further stigmatization of these groups, since they foster an impression that these groups are "to blame" for the epidemic. Moreover, such risk groups have in most cases no clearly defined identity and their members would not readily identify themselves as sex workers or homosexuals and so forth.

- The concept of risk groups has increasingly been expanded to "risk behaviour" (e.g. unprotected sexual intercourse). This was supposed to avoid limitation to certain groups of persons and their stigmatization.

- In addition, most HIV prevention programmes first concentrated on reducing the immediate risk of HIV infection by bringing about change in sexual behaviour. However, it proved difficult to achieve and maintain these behaviour changes: the "risk" approach did not take sufficiently into account the fact that behaviour is often not rationally determined (which is particularly true of sexual behaviour), and that people cannot implement what they have recognized as correct if they do not have the means to make self-determined decisions (Piot and Coll-Seck 2001). A few examples of this:

  - Sex-specific roles and power relations mean that women cannot successfully negotiate condom use.
  - Violence in the domestic sphere, in forced prostitution or in war prevents women and children from determining their sexual behaviour.
  - Dependence among drug users and criminalization of drug use result in the sharing of injection equipment, thus significantly increasing the HIV risk.

- The concept of vulnerability has been increasingly used. Vulnerable for HIV infection are people who, due to limited self-determination in social, sexual and other areas, have an increased risk of HIV infection: women, children, CSWs, homosexuals, young people, drug users, migrants, ethnic minorities and poor people. Vulnerability also relates to the higher susceptibility of these groups for the negative social effects of the epidemic: children, for example, are especially affected here.

- The Ecumenical Advocacy Alliance (2001a) says that vulnerable population groups require special attention, sympathy, trust and accompaniment. The social, economic and psychological structures which create and maintain vulnerability must be changed so that people attain greater control over their risk behaviour.

> The concept of vulnerability takes into account the limited self-determination in risk behaviour for HIV infection and the increased susceptibility for the effects of AIDS.

3.2 MIGRATION AND MOBILITY

- Many poor countries have a large number of people who, for varying reasons, migrate or are very mobile: truck drivers, CSWs, seasonal

> Migrants and mobile populations have an increased risk of HIV infection.

workers, traders, members of the military and so on. Urbanization contributes to further mobility.

- Migrants often change their sexual behaviour to a higher-risk one with several sexual partners and commercial sex. In the cities, the extended family no longer exists and/or is unable to function, so that traditional behaviour patterns and social control mechanisms are less active. Migrants and people who are mobile therefore have a higher risk of getting infected with HIV at the places where they stay and then taking the infection back home, often without even knowing it.

> For Southern Africa, migration represents an essential factor enhancing the spread of HIV.

- For the countries in Southern Africa, migration and the related life in single-sex hostels and disruption of families represent an essential factor promoting the spread of HIV. Some migrants (e.g. mineworkers) generally live in accommodation only for men, and prostitution is frequent in such an environment. Every year, seasonal workers are away from their home regions for months at a time. From South Africa and elsewhere it is reported that many women fear the return of their men from their work, because of the risk that they will bring HIV with them.

- In many Asian countries and elsewhere many women migrate in search of work. It is even more difficult for them to find adequate living and working conditions than it is for men. This makes them susceptible to sexual exploitation, and they thus have a high risk of HIV infection.

- Truck drivers were one of the first population groups to be affected by HIV. They are still very vulnerable to HIV infection due to their mobility and long absence from their families.

- Migrants and mobile population groups are also vulnerable since they have less access to information about HIV and care in the event of falling sick.

3.3 Wars, conflicts and refugees

- The crises, wars and conflicts existing in many countries are characterized by the collapse of traditional structures and a worsening of medical care and nutrition. These factors promote HIV transmission through increased vulnerability. For example, it is estimated that more than 3 million people have died in the Democratic Republic of Congo in recent years. The main causes of death were the accompanying consequences of war, such as malnutrition, violence, illness and AIDS.

> Due to mobility and negative male role patterns, members of the military run a greater risk of infecting themselves and others with HIV.

- HIV prevalence is especially high among members of the military. Due to their high mobility and negative male role patterns, members of the military contribute to the spread of HIV and are also themselves exposed to an increased risk of infection. The military, moreover, is often not adequately targeted by HIV prevention.

- In war, rape is employed as a "strategic" means, as has been the case in the DR Congo. In Rwanda, 80 per cent of all women who during the genocide were raped and then had themselves tested for HIV were found to be HIV-positive (UNHCR 2001).

- Also in Rwanda, before the genocide, the HIV prevalence was 10 per cent in the cities and 1 per cent in the rural areas. In 1997 it was 11 per cent in both urban and rural areas (UNAIDS 2002).

- Many African countries have accepted large refugee populations from neighbouring countries. Because traditional structures are destroyed and they generally do not have a secure income, refugees and internally displaced persons run a high risk of HIV infection. This is especially true for young girls and women, who exchange sex for housing, food, etc. Moreover, refugees are generally not integrated into national HIV prevention programmes. Finally, in the event of falling ill, they have limited access to adequate care and treatment.
- HIV/AIDS is often not adequately addressed in emergency situations, since it is thought that there are more pressing problems to be resolved. In light of the fact that emergency situations increase vulnerability and therefore HV transmission, it is vital to incorporate HIV prevention and treatment in programmes addressing humanitarian crises and war situations.

3.4 TRAFFICKING IN HUMAN BEINGS AND SEX TRADE

- Organized trafficking in human beings is increasing throughout the world. Africa, Asia and Eastern Europe are especially affected. Children are sold as servants or slaves in the domestic sphere and women and children are sold into sexual exploitation.
- Prostitution with children is increasing throughout the world, due in part to fears of HIV infection. It is widely assumed that children are "HIV-free".
- People affected by this are particularly vulnerable to HIV infection.
- The European states also have a responsibility here, since many of the women and children in the sex trade are brought to Europe. Through advocacy and lobbying one can combat the trafficking in human beings which is forcing many women into prostitution. An awareness of the interconnections between human rights, prostitution and HIV transmission must be created.

> Lobbying should be undertaken against trafficking in human beings and sex tourism.

3.5 COMMERCIAL SEX WORK

- A special target group in HIV programmes are commercial sex workers (CSWs), since frequently they have relatively high HIV infection rates due to numerous, mostly unprotected, sexual contacts.
- The group of CSWs is not homogeneous, however, but instead includes women whose lives differ from one another: women who earn their livelihood by prostitution; women who are forced by poverty to exchange sex for money or other favours (so-called transactional sex); sex work; forced prostitution and slavery.
- Even with "voluntary" prostitution, one must always look into living circumstances. In India, 50 per cent of CSWs are under 18 years of age, and 20 per cent are younger than 15. Many CSWs are subjected to sexual violence, which substantially increases the risk of HIV infection. In a study in Bangladesh, two-thirds of CSWs indicated that they had been raped in the last year. In Nepal, HIV prevalence among CSWs varied

> CSWs themselves, their clients and their partners must all be protected against HIV infection. As part of this effort, programmes must protect and promote the human rights of women.

between 1 per cent and 50 per cent, depending on whether and in what area of India they had worked. Among the 30 per cent of CSWs who were forced to go to India, an HIV infection was three times more likely than among those who had not been forced (UNICEF/UNAIDS/WHO 2002).

- Education and prevention must have the objective of protecting the women and their male partners, and thus also preventing the HIV infection from being passed on to others. CSWs are generally more willing to use condoms than their clients, but do not have the means to insist on condom use for fear of violence or loss of income. It is therefore vital to address male clients. This is neglected in many programmes, since it is found that male clients are difficult to reach.

- HIV/AIDS programmes should not result in even more pressure and violence being exercised against women and children in sex work.

> HIV/AIDS programmes should not result in more pressure and violence being exercised against women and children in sex work.

- Most programmes do not put prostitution as such into question. However, a prime objective of interventions should be to empower women so that they can pursue some other employment. With regard to men, one must seek to ensure that they respect the human dignity of women.

- Although sex tourism can facilitate the spread of HIV, there is scarce data on this. It urgently needs to be addressed in the rich countries.

3.6 INJECTING DRUG USE

- Injecting drug use in which needles, syringes and other injection equipment are shared between different users and used repeatedly entails an extremely high risk of HIV infection, if one or several users are HIV infected.

- Injecting drug users are frequently a neglected group in HIV prevention. More often than not they are regarded as a relatively closed group and stigmatized. Since drug use is generally illegal, those affected fear criminal prosecution and therefore rarely turn to prevention programmes.

> Harm-reduction programmes (including needle exchange) are effective in preventing HIV and are therefore urgently required among injecting drug users.

- Harm-reduction programmes have proven their value internationally and are scientifically recognized. They include methadone substitution for heroin-injecting users, decriminalization of drug consumption, needle exchange programmes and rehabilitation. However, so far, such programmes have only been implemented on a limited scale.

- In the almost complete absence of such programmes, the HIV epidemic in the states of Eastern Europe and of the Russian Federation, for example, is spreading among injecting drug users and via the heterosexual route to the rest of the population. The implementation of appropriate programmes is vital for effective HIV prevention.

- In many African countries very little is known about injecting drug use, and corresponding studies are lacking. However, many large cities are gaining increasing significance as centres for the international drug trade, and illicit drugs are being brought into the countries and sold.

3.7 Men who have sex with men (MSM)

- MSM (homosexuals) are on the whole a neglected group in most developing countries in HIV prevention activities. Homosexual behaviour is frequently stigmatized, so HIV prevention is made a great deal more difficult in this area.
- The number of sexual partners in this group is often high, while the use of condoms is low.
- Men who have sex with men often have sex with women as well. This must be taken into consideration in prevention efforts.
- Homosexual behaviour is often not spoken about and regarded as a taboo. For example, in a survey in the Philippines, 15 per cent of men surveyed acknowledged having had sexual intercourse with another man in the past year. In Cambodia, the HIV infection rate among MSMs is 15 per cent. For Africa, there are no official data on homosexual behaviour among men and its contribution to HIV transmission. One suspects that homosexual practices play a certain role in several countries. They are especially widespread in prisons.

> In many countries, homosexual behaviour is stigmatized and also in part criminalized, which makes HIV prevention more difficult.

4. Gender equity

4.1 VULNERABILITY TO HIV INFECTION

- "Gender" is defined as the expectations and norms within a society with regard to appropriate male and female behaviour and roles, which attribute to women and men different access to status and power, including resources and decision-making power.
- The spread of HIV/AIDS is to a great extent driven by gender inequity that infringes on women's social and sexual rights. HIV/AIDS infections are increasing disproportionately among women.
- Gender norms have a significant impact on the risk and vulnerability of people to becoming infected with HIV and influence the effects which HIV/AIDS has on people. Every analysis of the HIV epidemic must therefore also integrate the gender perspective.
- Interventions to fight HIV/AIDS must be gender sensitive: they must take into account their effects with respect to women, men and gender equity.
- In general, women have greater vulnerability to HIV infection. Unequal power positions in social life also manifest themselves in sexual relationships. Women generally have fewer possibilities than their male partners to determine whether and under what conditions sexual intercourse will occur, whether condoms are used (safer sex), etc.
- Women generally have little access to information about sexuality, reproductive health (including HIV/AIDS) and the corresponding means, such as condoms. The illiteracy rate is often higher among women than among men. Women in rural areas are especially disadvantaged.
- In many societies, girls become sexually active at an earlier age than males. They are generally especially disadvantaged, above all when society expects that girls should be ignorant in the area of sexuality.
- For many women, above all in Africa, the greatest risk factor for HIV infection is that they live in a monogamous relationship in which the husband has more than one partner, and at the same time they are not in a position to either refuse sex or insist on the use of condoms. Their economic dependency impels them to fear the consequences of leaving their relationship even more than the risk of HIV infection.
- There are several reasons why it is often impossible for a woman to insist on the use of condoms: she runs the risk of appearing unfaithful if she presses to have condoms used within marriage; the desire for children runs counter to the use of condoms; a sexual relationship is not the place where one "negotiates" condom use; it is often the fear of a violent response from her partner which dissuades her from insisting that condoms be used.
- Frequently, women are also de facto unequal under the law. In many countries their property rights are restricted. Often, they have no right to the property of the deceased husband, or the inheritance is taken away from them by members of the family ("property grabbing"). Widows are economically and socially disadvantaged and can be forced to exchange

sex for money or other things in order to ensure their own survival and that of their children. This exposes these women (and their sexual partners) to an increased risk of HIV infection.
- Certain traditions can contribute to the vulnerability of women. In several areas it was traditional that a man marry the widow of his deceased brother (wife inheritance, levirate marriage) or that he have sexual intercourse with her, in order to purify her (sexual cleansing). The custom of remarriage with the brother was originally conceived for the protection of widows against the loss of their land. The HIV epidemic means that in these cases the participants run a risk of being infected with HIV.
- The social and economic independence of women must be promoted in order to contain the HIV epidemic. In the short term, this can be achieved through income-generating measures, small-scale loans, etc. Over the long term, education and training must be allowed to take effect, and government policies designed to promote gender equity have to be put in place and enforced.

> Fighting HIV also entails improving the social and economic position of women.

4.2 GIRLS AND YOUNG WOMEN

- In many African countries in the age group 15–24 years, 2–8 times more women are HIV-infected than men (Laga et al. 2001). This finding is encountered at all HIV prevalence rates, and is more pronounced in urban areas than rural ones. The following graph shows HIV prevalences in several African countries (source: UNAIDS 2002):

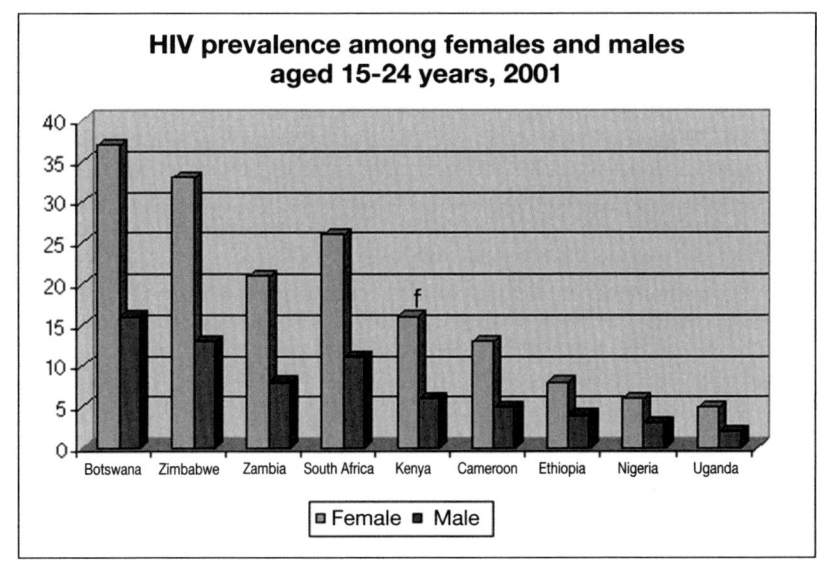

- In the higher age groups (over 30), the relationship reverses, and generally HIV infection rates are higher among men than among women.
- These differences in HIV prevalence among young people are not caused by the extent of sexual activity. Studies have shown that boys commence

> In Africa, young girls and women 15–24 years of age have 2–8 times higher infection rates than men of the same age. An important reason for this is that young girls frequently have (unprotected) sexual intercourse with older men, who for their part have a higher probability of being infected with HIV.

sexual activity just as early as girls, and that moreover they have more partners before marriage than girls of the same age. This means that even a higher level of sexual activity among boys does not lead to the same rapid increase in HIV prevalence as among girls (Laga et al. 2001).

- The reason for the higher prevalence among girls is rather that, in many countries, young girls tend to have sexual intercourse with older men who, for their part, have a higher risk of being infected with HIV ("sugar daddies"). In these relationships, sex frequently takes place in exchange for financial or other favours, and condoms are almost never used. Moreover, the girls also have sex with boys of their own age, in order to find a potential husband. Here, too, condom use is low (Gregson et al. 2002). As the economic situation worsens, sexual relationships between young girls and older men will further increase.
- Older men often seek girls as sexual partners on the assumption that the latter are HIV-free, or even that sexual intercourse with a young girl or a child (a "virgin") will cure them of their own HIV infection.
- The unequal balance of social power in these relationships makes it very unlikely that girls can negotiate for protected sexual intercourse (safer sex). The risk also increases with sexual intercourse which leads to injuries and bleeding, as in the case with forced sex or defloration.
- The girls run a high risk of being infected with HIV by their older sexual partners. They can also infect these partners, as well as their future husbands and children.
- Young girls also have a higher rate of untreated sexually transmitted infections than do boys of the same age (above all, Herpes Simplex virus infections), which promote HIV transmission.
- Prevention programmes should instruct young girls about sexuality and reproductive health. This should begin before the girls become sexually active. The girls must develop an awareness of their risk and be provided with the necessary skills to implement what they have learned and not yield to the pressure of same-age or older sexual partners. Girls must acquire skills which empower them to be economically more independent and not rely on financial support.
- School attendance on the part of girls must be promoted and, where possible, made free of charge. School attendance delays the beginning of sexual activity. It is particularly tragic that many girls enter into a sexual relationship with an older man in order to secure their school fees.
- Virginity and abstinence before marriage should be presented as positive values for boys as well.
- However, it may nevertheless be necessary to establish or increase girls' access to condoms. Girls generally have no money available for condoms, they are stigmatized if they purchase condoms, and they lack the confidence to buy them and talk about them with their partners.
- AIDS programmes which wish to protect young girls and women against HIV infection must also be directed at men, and at society in general:
  - Myths about curing HIV through sexual intercourse with a young girl must be combated.

Programmes to protect girls from sexual exploitation and HIV infection must also address men. The churches have important work to do in creating awareness within communities, and should critically analyse their own attitudes.

- • "Demand reduction" must be achieved by instructing and educating men. Sexual intercourse with a young girl must cease to be socially acceptable (UNICEF 2001b).
- The churches have an important mission and great potential here. Through their access to young people, and particularly girls, they can implement adequate prevention programmes. Through their access to adult men within their communities, they can create awareness for responsible sexual behaviour. It is necessary that churches critically analyse their own role and attitudes with respect to the problem.

4.3 Gender-based and sexual violence

- For physiological reasons, the risk of HIV transmission is much higher for a woman if the sexual encounter includes violence. The trauma leads to bleeding and therefore carries a higher risk of HIV infection. Moreover, perpetrators of sexual violence are more likely to be HIV infected.
- Awareness of the links between sexual violence and HIV transmission is however just emerging.
- Many girls and women encounter sexual violence in everyday life: in their families, communities, and within institutions such as schools, where violence is exercised by male classmates and teachers against schoolgirls.
- In war and in conflict, women and girls are especially vulnerable and exposed to the risk of sexual violence. Alongside the risk of unwanted pregnancies and sexually transmitted infections, the danger of HIV infection is particularly high.
- The genital mutilation of girls practised in some countries ("circumcision") increases the risk of HIV infection through the practice itself, which under certain circumstances is implemented with the same instruments on several girls, and through the subsequent greater vulnerability during sexual intercourse later in life.
- Gender-based violence is difficult to challenge, since it is a particular taboo in communities where women and girls who suffer from it are often stigmatized rather than empowered.

Sexual violence (in families and institutions, in war, in prostitution, etc.) increases the risk of HIV infection.

4.4 Impact of HIV/AIDS on women

- The HIV epidemic contributes to the generally already substantial workload of women and girls. Women – and increasingly girls as well – bear the greatest share of care in families and communities:
  - • They care for the increasing number of orphans.
  - • They do volunteer work in home-based care.
  - • They care for the chronically sick at home and frequently also in hospital.
- AIDS-related deaths of other family members and impoverishment increase the workload of women (e.g. in the fields).

The HIV epidemic increases the workload of women and girls: through caring for the chronically sick, the death of family members and impoverishment.

- Impoverishment through AIDS in turn increases vulnerability to HIV infection, by diminishing the economic basis of women, which exposes them to the risk of sexual exploitation.
- The assumption that the breadwinner – and thus the decision-maker – in families is a man underestimates and undermines the position and significance of women, and is thus counter-productive. Women often contribute significantly to family income. Women work in the subsistence economy and thus are primarily responsible for producing food for their families. This is further strengthened by the HIV/AIDS epidemic: in Africa, 70 per cent of rural households are headed by women, either because there is no husband or he is away for long periods (e.g. due to labour migration).
- Women often suffer a double stigma of living with HIV/AIDS and being female.
- Education of girls has a stimulating effect on entire societies. A higher educational level for women reduces the average number of children and improves the state of health of families. However, in many developing countries, the educational system is inadequate and the proportion of girls attending school is relatively low. AIDS further disadvantages girls:
  - The death of teachers reduces the educational opportunities overall, thus also those of girls.
  - School fees often represent a significant burden for the meagre family budget, and girls are frequently the first to have to leave school.
  - By assuming the responsibility for caring for sick family members as well as younger siblings, girls can no longer attend school.
- The future prospects of girls are limited by inadequate school education. Since they have fewer chances of becoming economically and socially independent later, they have an increased risk of HIV infection. Girls who are orphans are especially affected.

> *AIDS substantially restricts educational opportunities for girls.*

4.5 MEN

4.5.1 Addressing and involving men

- Gender is not about women's issues only, as it has sometimes been understood. Focusing on women's empowerment is critical, but it has to be complemented by involving and empowering men and changing male attitudes, stereotypes and behaviours that further the spread of HIV.
- Many AIDS interventions have identified women and girls as target groups. However, in order that men protect themselves and their female partners against HIV infection, it is necessary to address men directly and promote their responsible sexual behaviour.
  - Conventional male-role stereotypes, which regard multiple sexual partners, sexual violence or unprotected sexual intercourse as proof of manhood, must be critically analysed and corrected.
  - Most volunteer AIDS work is carried out by women. Men have to be more actively involved in the fight against AIDS, as volunteers, agents of change, etc.

> *Conventional male role stereotypes must be critically analysed and corrected. Powerful men (e.g. in institutions) must not use their power to expose women and girls to the risk of HIV infection.*

- - Men in institutions (military, police, teachers, church) must not exploit their socially more powerful position to persuade or compel girls and women to engage in sexual activities, and to expose themselves, their families and the affected women to the risk of HIV transmission.
  - Commercial sex should not be viewed as an expression of sexuality, but rather as the treatment of another person as a commodity and as exploitation of an unequal power relationship.
- Men should also be encouraged to play a more active role in caring for the chronically sick within families and communities, so as to relieve the women in these tasks and to contribute to reducing HIV stigma.
- In many programmes it is necessary to address women and men separately. In discussions and education about sexuality and AIDS, men and women must have a free space in which they can discuss matters without the other sex being involved. Only after such a process should discussions in mixed groups take place.
- HIV programmes which target both men and boys should not replace programmes aimed at women and girls; rather, they should complement them.

> HIV programmes which target both men and boys should not replace programmes aimed at women and girls; rather, they should complement them.

4.5.2 Vulnerability of men and boys

- Paying attention to the gender aspects of AIDS also means taking into account men's vulnerability to HIV infection:
  - It appears that the taboos associated with AIDS are often even more pronounced for men, so that generally more women than men visit AIDS counselling centres. Men should be strongly encouraged to make use of these resources.
  - Sexual role behaviour which tolerates or encourages multiple sexual partners for men also increases men's risk of HIV infection.
  - Migrants are vulnerable because frequently familial and marital bonds are loosened and the possibility of riskier sexual behaviour (changing partners, no condom use) increases.
  - Young men are often better informed about sexuality and reproductive health than young women. However, they are frequently insufficiently informed to protect themselves against HIV infection. Gender role behaviour can then further impede the adequate acquisition of information, since admitting to ignorance in this area does not accord with the male role cliché.
  - The use of alcohol and drugs, which in many societies forms part of the male role, contributes to greater vulnerability.

> Men are in many respects vulnerable to HIV infection, conditioned by male role definitions.

5. Children

5.1 Children living with HIV

In 2001, 3 million children were living with HIV throughout the world.

- The table shows global and regional estimates of the HIV epidemic among children (< 15 years) for the year 2001 (source: UNAIDS 2002):

Region	Children living with HIV	New infections	AIDS deaths
Sub-Saharan Africa	2,600,000	700,000	520,000
Northern Africa & Middle East	35,000	12,000	6,000
South Asia & Southeast Asia	220,000	60,000	42,000
East Asia & Pacific	3,000	3,000	1,600
Latin America	40,000	10,000	5,000
Caribbean	20,000	7,000	6,800
Eastern Europe & Central Asia	15,000	1,000	<100
Western Europe	5,000	<500	<100
North America	10,000	<500	<100
Australia & New Zealand	<200	<100	<100
Total	**3,000,000**	**800,000**	**580,000**

In 2001, 2.4 million children were living with HIV in sub-Saharan Africa.

- At the end of 2001, 2.6 million children below age 15 were living with HIV in Africa, and 520,000 children died of HIV during the course of that year. In this region, 700,000 children were newly infected in 2001, generally through mother-to-child transmission (UNAIDS 2002).
- Most children who are infected with HIV through vertical transmission die during the first two years of life if they do not have access to antiretroviral drugs. Some children survive until the age of 5 years or even longer, depending on the food situation, access to medical care and other factors. Improved access to antiretroviral drugs in poor countries would also be of benefit for HIV-infected children, since these drugs are also available for children.

5.2 Orphans

AIDS has created 14 million orphans around the world.

- More than 14 million children below the age of 15 have lost one or both parents due to AIDS, 11 million of them in sub-Saharan Africa. It is expected that by the year 2010 this number will have risen to more than 25 million, perhaps to more than 40 million (UNAIDS/UNICEF 2002; UNFPA 2002).
- For example, in South Africa, 13 per cent of all 2–14 year-old children have lost either one or both parents (HSRC 2002).

- The increasing number of orphans generates serious consequences for the affected societies. HIV/AIDS is the main cause of the increase in child mortality in many countries. For example, in Zimbabwe, 70 per cent of all deaths among children under 5 years of age are AIDS related (UNAIDS 2001a).
- Although the fertility of populations is decreasing due to AIDS-related deaths among young adults in the severely affected countries, population growth will probably remain positive. Therefore, a relatively small number of economically active adults will have to provide for a large number of dependents – children and older people. Adequate care and education are then no longer guaranteed.
- Inadequate socialization may lead to an increase in crime, prostitution, and to a shortage of skilled workers in all social areas, with a subsequent decline in economic growth, impoverishment, etc.
- In countries with high HIV prevalence, the future prospects of all children are significantly limited. HIV is one of the greatest obstacles to the realization of children's rights (UNICEF 2001c).

> In countries with high HIV prevalence, the future prospects of *all* children are limited.

- Although orphans are often especially disadvantaged, in the developing countries many children do not have what is necessary to survive. For example, 42 per cent of children in Zambia suffer from chronic malnutrition, which leads to stunted growth and prevents them from attaining their full intellectual and mental potential in adulthood (UNICEF 2000a).
- One therefore speaks generally of orphans/vulnerable children (OVC). They are disadvantaged in many respects: they often experience a lack of care from their parents, inadequate schooling, etc.
- Children are traumatized when one parent or both parents die of AIDS. When they are accepted into a new family, they sometimes experience the same fate again.

> If enough other adult family members are no longer available, orphans must themselves head households and take care of their younger brothers and sisters, or they are looked after by grandparents.

- Due to the extreme increase in the number of orphans and those dying of AIDS, in many places the extended families which in traditional societies cared for orphans are no longer in a position to meet these demands.
- After the death of the parents, in the event of the unavailability of other adult caretakers, children – often as early as 8–10 years of age – are forced to look after their younger siblings and themselves (child-headed households). In Zambia there are approximately 130,000 households (i.e. around 15 per cent of all households) which are headed by children (Kelly 1999).
- Many orphans are cared for by their grandparents, who normally would themselves be dependent on care from their adult children, since in poor countries there are generally no provisions for old age through pensions and the like. Moreover, the grandparents are exhausted from a long working life, and finally they have been psychologically strained by the death of their own children from AIDS.
- Households run by children and grandparents lack the necessary capacity and resources to guarantee an adequate food supply, education and training for the children.
- A study in western Kenya found an exponential increase in the number of orphans. Most of them could not pay school fees and suffered from a

lack of food, clothing and healthcare. The traditional system of relatives had supported the children in many ways but, due to the scarcity of resources, it was no longer in a position to deal adequately with the situation (Nyadhemba et al. 2001).
– Orphans, above all girls, frequently have a heightened risk of (sexual) exploitation and therefore also of HIV infection.

5.3 STREET CHILDREN

> Street children are especially vulnerable to HIV infection.

– Street children are children who either no longer have a home or prefer to live on the street because conditions in their homes have become intolerable for them. Most of them are boys; however, an unknown number of girls are also affected.
– Street children are found above all in the major cities; however, their number is also increasing in rural areas. According to estimates, there are tens of thousands of street children in cities like Nairobi and Lusaka.
– Boys and girls living on the street have an increased risk of (sexual) violence and drug consumption, and are therefore especially vulnerable to HIV infection.

5.4 SEXUAL EXPLOITATION

– The spread of HIV/AIDS is tied up in a complex structure with the sexual exploitation of children. Orphans run an especially high risk of sexual exploitation, because they have lost the protection of their families. Every year, 1 million children are forced into the sex trade, where they are especially vulnerable to becoming infected with HIV (UNICEF 2001b).

> In several regions it is believed that HIV can be cured through sexual intercourse with a virgin.

– In several countries, such as South Africa, it is believed that HIV can be cured through sexual intercourse with a virgin. The South African President Thabo Mbeki has called for a stop to the wave of rapes of babies and children, which are often carried out by infected men in the belief that it will cure their HIV infection (Mbeki 2001).

5.5 EDUCATION ON SEX AND SEXUALITY

– It is often argued that it is difficult or inadvisable to speak with children before puberty about sexuality. Counter-arguments, however, show that sex education for children is important:
  - Throughout the world, children are increasingly confronted with sexuality (mostly as a commodity) via video, advertisements, television, etc.
  - What young people learn about sexuality from their peers generally does not promote the development of responsible sexual behaviour. Therefore, adults must convey appropriate messages to children and young people early on.
  - In reality, many young people are sexually active. In many countries, there are pregnancies – partially through forced sexual intercourse –

of 9–10 year-old girls. In Zambia, for example, one-half of all girls under the age of 18 either already have a child or are pregnant. Thus it would seem inappropriate not to talk with young people about sexuality.

- It has been repeatedly demonstrated that sex education does not lead to earlier sexual behaviour but, quite the contrary, delays sexual activity and leads to more responsible sexual behaviour. Long-lasting behaviour patterns (including postponement of the beginning of sexual activity) are learned in the period between 10 and 14 years of age. Establishing such behaviour patterns in children is easier than changing high-risk behaviour later (UNICEF/UNAIDS/WHO 2002).

> Sex education does not lead to early sexual behaviour; on the contrary, it serves to delay sexual activity. Appropriate messages from adults must therefore be communicated to children at an early age.

– Many programmes and initiatives have started to target primary school children and children of similar ages in HIV prevention.

5.6 Care and support

– The preference in the care of orphans should be to place them within their own (extended) family. If this is impossible because the extended family cannot be identified or the death of adult family members has exhausted the capacities of families to accept orphans, attempts should be made to find a foster family.

– There are many examples of families that have incorporated children from other families. Were this not the case, the problem in countries hardest hit by HIV would be even worse than it already is. Many families are pushed to the limits of their resilience and beyond in their efforts to care for orphans. They therefore need support to care and be responsible for children.

– Many AIDS programmes have components for supporting orphans. For example, home care programmes support orphans and other needy children with food, school fees and school uniforms. Programmes which support orphans in families should not selectively support these children alone, since non-orphans are also needy. Support should go to the entire family, whereby it should be guaranteed that the orphans also benefit appropriately.

– Orphans whose parents died of AIDS must not be discriminated against by identifying and stigmatizing them as "AIDS orphans". Also, other children – non-orphans or orphans for other reasons – should be included in care programmes, if they are in need:

- Not all children whose parents died of AIDS are especially vulnerable and, conversely, it is not necessarily the case that all other children and other orphans are not needy.

- For many orphans, the cause of death of the parents is not known. A positive HIV test of parents should not be made a prerequisite for including the child in a support programme, since this can lead to stigmatization.

- Children whose parents died of AIDS must not become the objects of positive discrimination, so that other children in need do not receive access to the service.

> As far as possible, orphans should be placed in a family. Families and communities need support in order to manage these tasks. Orphanages should only serve as a last resort, when all other options have been exhausted.

- Orphanages have substantial disadvantages: they are relatively cost-intensive, their long-term sustainability is generally uncertain, and the children are separated from their family environment. Orphanages can merely serve as a last resort when all other options have been exhausted.
- This can be the case, for example, when a temporary admission (e.g. in refugee situations) is necessary.

6. Young people

6.1 Impact on young people

- In 2001, 11.8 million young people between the ages of 15 and 24 were living with HIV. One-half of new HIV infections worldwide occur within this age group. 6,000 young people are infected with HIV every day. Only a fraction of the infected persons know of their HIV infection.
- Through its social and economic consequences, the HIV epidemic has an impact on the lives of all young people, since it limits the future prospects of HIV-negative young people as well.

> In 2001, throughout the world 11.8 million young people between the ages of 15 and 24 were living with HIV. Where the spread of HIV has been halted, it has been achieved primarily through a behaviour change among young people.

6.2 Knowledge on sexuality and AIDS

- Serious deficits still exist around the world in the information young people have about HIV. Although a majority have heard of HIV/AIDS, many do not know how HIV is spread and do not believe that they personally run any risk of becoming infected. For example, two-thirds of the young people in a study in Botswana thought that they could recognize, merely on the basis of appearance, whether or not a person is infected with HIV. Even young people who know something about HIV often do not protect themselves against infection because they lack the necessary skills, support and resources to behave appropriately.
- Wherever the spread of HIV has been stopped, it has been achieved primarily through a behaviour change among young people and young adults. It has been shown that young people can responsibly protect themselves and others if they receive appropriate support.
- For most people, sexual activity begins in adolescence. Recent studies in Brazil, Hungary and Kenya have shown that more than one-quarter of the boys surveyed indicated that they had had sex before their fifteenth birthday.
- Young people who begin with sexual activity early have sex more frequently with high-risk partners, have several partners more often, and use condoms less frequently. Delaying the age of first sexual activity can significantly protect young people from HIV infection (UNICEF/UNAIDS/WHO 2002).

> Young people have significant information deficits concerning HIV/AIDS. In addition, most young people lack the necessary resources and skills to effectively protect themselves against infection.

> Postponing the first sexual activity can significantly protect young people from HIV infection.

6.3 HIV/AIDS education

- It has been shown that sex education does not, as is sometimes asserted, lead to an earlier start of sexual activity among children and young people, but rather, on the contrary, to beginning activities later and to dealing with sexuality more responsibly.
- AIDS education should be integrated into health and sex education, but it should also be dealt with as an independent theme. Children and young people must grow up with an awareness that HIV/AIDS is a reality in their lives. Programmes should help children and young people to delay the commencement of sexual activity. They should effectively protect

> The objective of sex and AIDS education is to lead young people to engage in responsible sexual behaviour.

– young people against HIV infection, other sexually transmitted infections and unwanted pregnancies.

– Sexuality must not be dealt with merely in medical and biological terms, but rather must be seen in the context of its significance for the lives of young people. The objective of such an education is to lead young people to deal responsibly with their sexuality.

– Many young people experience peer pressure to engage in sexual activity. Here one must deploy strategies which strengthen the self-confidence of young people, above all that of girls, and give them the necessary assertiveness.

> Initiation rites can be an approach for educating young people about HIV.

– In many societies, parents traditionally did not speak with their children openly about sexuality. Education about sexuality, marriage, partnership, etc. was handled by other adults. It occurred partially through initiation rites, which in many societies were a stable component of the introduction into adult life for girls and boys in early adolescence. These rites taught the responsibilities incumbent upon an adult member of the community: housekeeping, respect for elders, the relations of the partners in marriage, etc. However, in many societies this custom has been abandoned over the years.

– In some places, there is an attempt by churches and others to rediscover these traditions and to incorporate HIV/AIDS into the "curriculum" of initiations. This could be a promising approach for reaching young people (especially girls and those who do not attend school) in AIDS prevention.

> For most young people, abstinence is the preferable option. But HIV interventions should not insist on a single strategy: they must take into account the reality of young people's lives, in which sexual activity frequently plays a role.

– HIV prevention messages are often contradictory. Some programmes communicate that HIV infections can only be prevented by condoms; in others, condoms are not allowed under any circumstances. For most young people, abstinence is certainly the option which is to be preferred and which also offers the greatest protection against HIV infection. However, it is problematic when HIV interventions insist on a single strategy and ignore the reality of young people's lives, in which sexual activity often plays a role. If the uppermost objective of HIV prevention is that young people not use condoms, this can result in young people simply having sexual intercourse without condoms.

– HIV prevention often treats sexuality only from the perspective of group pressure, exchange of sex for money, and sexual violence. However, sexuality has a positive value – and not only in the lives of young people: youth is the time when one falls in love and seeks a life partner. That sexual activity can bring about death is especially difficult for young people to understand and integrate into their lives. If HIV prevention programmes are to be credible and effective, these interrelations must be taken into account.

– Interventions must be targeted at all young people, not only to those with a perceived "high risk".

> Young people must be responsibly integrated into all interventions which concern them.

– Many programmes for young people are not very effective because they are conceived and implemented exclusively by adults. Young people must be responsibly integrated into all aspects of AIDS interventions which concern them (i.e. the development, implementation and evaluation of programmes). Only in this way can it be guaranteed that they assume responsibility (ownership) for the programmes, that the form and content of the communication are well-adapted for young people, and that the programmes are effective and sustainable.

- Adults, above all parents, teachers, clergy and other educators, bear an enormous responsibility in HIV prevention. Taboo subjects and unpleasant realities, such as sexual violence, must be addressed. Churches and communities should integrate sex and AIDS education into the programmes of their youth groups, children's groups, confirmation groups, etc. In Zambia, for example, there are Anti-AIDS Clubs in many schools, where sexuality and AIDS are discussed and role plays are performed on the theme.

- Health facilities can make a decisive contribution to educating young people about sexual health, including HIV. To achieve this they must be "youth friendly": they must not turn away and stigmatize young people, they must ensure confidentiality and, when appropriate, they should provide access to condoms (Mwakagile et al. 2001; UNICEF/UNAIDS/WHO 2002).

> Churches and communities should integrate HIV education into their youth groups, children's groups, confirmation groups, Sunday schools, etc.

7. Socio-economic context

7.1 Poverty, development and socio-economic impact

The social and economic impact of the HIV epidemic is serious. However, there is still insufficient data on this complex subject.

– The impact of the HIV/AIDS epidemic is already serious and it is going to get worse. It is difficult to forecast with precision, however, because there is still too little data and the problem has not yet attracted the attention it deserves.

– In the high-prevalence countries, all people are affected by the epidemic. They are either themselves infected with HIV or are affected as members of the family, survivors, orphans and members of the community (people infected with and affected by HIV).

– Poverty fosters the spread of HIV and exacerbates the impact on individuals, communities and societies. Globally, HIV/AIDS is a disease associated with poverty: it disproportionately affects people in poor countries and the poorer population groups within the rich industrialized countries. The Ecumenical Advocacy Alliance (2001a) has invited churches to highlight AIDS as a poverty-related illness.

People living in poverty are even further impoverished by HIV/AIDS. They have a higher risk of becoming infected with HIV, which then goes on to affect the following generation (e.g. through a lack of schooling).

– People who live in poverty are further impoverished by HIV, since wage-earners die, savings are consumed and expenses for medical treatment and funerals increase. A vicious circle develops: the poor have less access to treatment and care in the event of chronic sickness; they lose their already low incomes and thus have even less access to resources. This increases their risk of HIV infection. The following generation is also affected: due to lack of education and subsequent lower social status, girls are more susceptible for commercial sex and other situations which increase their vulnerability to HIV.

– The kinds of social security systems which are widely available in the Western industrialized nations either do not exist at all in the developing countries, or only in rudimentary form, so that the social effects of HIV on individuals and families are not alleviated.

– Many poor countries depend on a small number of highly qualified specialists in key areas. In the most severely affected countries, large numbers of these well-educated people are dying. For example, 58 per cent of the deaths in Kenya's Agricultural Ministry are AIDS related (FAO 2001). Vital services, such as the healthcare system and schools, are being disrupted by HIV. At the same time, the HIV epidemic is placing greater demands on these services, while the traditional security systems, such as extended families, are being limited in their ability to function.

– Through the chronic illness and death of people in their most productive years, AIDS seriously affects societies by undermining social cohesion, threatening social and political stability and reducing the country's economic efficiency and growth. The epidemic substantially slows economic growth: in the 1990s AIDS reduced per capita growth in Africa by 0.8 per cent. It is estimated that by 2020, in the most heavily affected countries, growth will be 20–40 per cent lower than it would be without AIDS (UNFPA 2002).

- The impact of HIV/AIDS strikes workers and their families, companies and entire economies. The epidemic is undermining the social and economic advances which were achieved in recent decades and threatens further progress (ILO 2001). Negative effects for industry and companies develop through the death of employees; additional expenditures for training; insurance and pension payments; absence of employees due to illness, caring for family members and burials; and reduction of the labour supply.
- A country's entire economy may be affected by a reduction in tax revenues, lower profitability and productivity and a lower savings–income ratio.
- These negative consequences in turn promote the further spread of HIV/AIDS, and thus also jeopardize prevention and treatment efforts.
- The threat posed by the long-term consequences of HIV/AIDS is present in any case. Even if HIV transmission was halted today, the social consequences would remain serious, conditioned by the high number of those who have already died and those already infected.

> HIV/AIDS negates the social and economic advances of the developing countries and threatens further progress.

7.2 Poverty and health

- The fact that poverty conditions disease has been acknowledged for many years. Yet disease also conditions poverty and underdevelopment: premature mortality and reduction of the average life expectancy of people in poor countries due to HIV/AIDS, malaria, tuberculosis, childhood diseases, malnutrition and maternal mortality are essentially responsible for the economic "underdevelopment" of these countries, and yet could be remedied with relatively simple health-related measures. This was the conclusion of the Commission on Macroeconomics and Health in their report published at the end of 2001. The Commission had been assigned to investigate the significance of health for economic development in poor countries.
- The above-mentioned illnesses lower labour productivity and lead to worsened school performances, and in this way have a negative effect on economic growth. Reduced life expectancy also leads to people saving less, thereby decreasing the resources available for investments. Moreover, countries with high HIV prevalence are less attractive for investors, which also hinders economic growth.
- The report of the Commission presented yet another basis for calculation, one which is perhaps the most meaningful, since it also takes the long-term consequences (of HIV and other diseases) into account. Every premature death leads to a loss of potential years of life, especially when it occurs among young people. Health economists call this phenomenon (including limitations due to periods of illness and handicaps) loss of Disability Adjusted Life Years (DALYs).
- HIV/AIDS causes the loss of very many DALYs (34.6 on average), due to the age structure of those affected. In this way, already in 1999 AIDS had caused sub-Saharan Africa to lose 11.7 per cent of its economic power. Economists have calculated that the economic loss per DALY amounts to three times the annual income. This makes sense if one

> In the severely affected countries, disease and death are causing the loss of many resources. The very stability of whole societies is being threatened, and poverty is increasing. These factors in turn promote the further spread of HIV.

> Disease conditions poverty and underdevelopment: premature mortality due to HIV/AIDS contributes to the underdevelopment of many countries.

considers that one breadwinner generally provides for several other persons as well, and that consumption behaviour and above all investment behaviour changes. Persons with a long life expectancy invest substantially more in areas with a promising future (e.g. training, provisions for old age, etc.).

– This calculation is important if one wants to estimate the cost-effectiveness of investing in fighting AIDS. By no means may an average per capita income be taken as a starting point for such calculations, as has usually happened. One life-year saved corresponds to at least three times the annual income (Commission on Macroeconomics and Health 2001).

7.3 AGRICULTURAL SECTOR AND FOOD SECURITY

> It is estimated that in Africa 25 per cent of the agricultural labour force will die of AIDS by 2020.

– More than two-thirds of the population in the countries most affected by HIV in Africa live in rural areas. Since 1987, 7 million agricultural workers have died of AIDS. It is estimated that by the year 2020 up to 25 per cent of the agricultural labour force will die of AIDS (i.e. 16 million people) if the epidemic continues in the way it has spread in the past (FAO 2001).

– A study in a rural area in Western Tanzania found that an HIV prevalence of 7 per cent of the adult population had a substantial impact on mortality among adults. Life expectancy was around 43 years. Furthermore, the mobility of household members before and after the death of a member was high: in 44 per cent of cases in which the head of the household died, the inhabitants left the house and the household was dissolved (Urassa et al. 2001).

– Rural communities are subject to high levels of stress due to HIV, since many HIV-infected persons return from the city to their native villages when they require care, as well as to die there.

– Because there is less access to information and health facilities in the countryside than in the city, people in rural areas have less information about how they can protect themselves against HIV infection and, in the event of falling sick, have less access to care and treatment.

– The food security of families, communities and states is already impaired and is increasingly threatened:

  - Agricultural workers, including in the subsistence economy, are being lost.
  - Care of sick relatives and orphans takes up time which then is no longer available for agricultural work.
  - Families sell their possessions in order to cover the costs of chronic disease, burials and the loss of workers.
  - People die before they can pass on their knowledge to the next generation.
  - Investments such as in irrigation and soil improvement projects are reduced.
  - Increasing amounts of grain are cultivated, which is less labour-intensive, but which also has less nutritional value.

- Cash crops are grown at the expense of crops for own consumption.
- Animals are sold and slaughtered in order to feed the sick and pay expenses.
- Diminishing revenues lead to a loss of purchasing power within the overall social context.

– Women are particularly affected, since their workload increases more than proportionally. After the death of their husbands they often find they have no right to the land. They are no longer able to produce sufficient food or earn enough money to buy seeds and food.

– Due to the inadequate food supply, the health of people (especially children) and their resistance to HIV diseases are further impaired.

– The lack of vitamins and trace elements (vitamins A, B, C, D, E, zinc and selenium) accelerates the progress of HIV/AIDS illness and under certain circumstances also leads to an increased transmission rate.

– The severe hunger catastrophe in several countries in Southern Africa during 2002 is closely interwoven with the HIV crisis. In the affected countries, over 1 million people have already died of AIDS, and almost 15 million are infected with HIV, many of whom are chronically ill or in a weakened condition. HIV/AIDS is likely to have a severe impact on future food security of whole countries if adequate interventions are not forthcoming.

> HIV reduces food security. An inadequate food supply in turn makes people more susceptible to HIV infection and aggravates the course of the disease, leading to an earlier death.

7.4 EDUCATION SECTOR

– Worldwide, 100 million children – 60 million of them girls – do not receive an elementary education. These children come predominantly from HIV/AIDS-affected communities, conflict and war zones, poor families and rural areas (UNICEF 2001a). AIDS reduces the number of children who attend school because:
- Families cannot afford to pay school fees.
- Families are destroyed.
- Children have to work in the house and fields, and care for the sick; or are engaged in income-generating activities.

– The lack of school education has negative consequences for the future of the affected children, and for society as a whole. In particular, when girls receive school education birth rates go down and the level of family health improves.

– AIDS also has an impact on the educational system by reducing the number of teachers and others active in the system, such as inspectors, administrative staff, etc. For example, in Zambia the death rate among teachers is 70 per cent higher than among the general adult population, and the number of teachers dying from AIDS is twice as high as the number of teachers completing their teacher training (Kelly 1999).

– The resources at the disposal of the educational sector have declined because tax revenues are falling as a result of HIV and resources are being redistributed. This means that fewer teachers can be trained and those who retire are not being replaced. In some areas, entire classes or

> AIDS leads to a reduction in the number of schoolgoing children by increasing poverty and reducing the number of teachers. This especially affects orphans and girls.

schools are being closed, which leads to a further decline in the numbers of pupils. The quality of education continues to worsen.

– Many communities which actively contributed resources to the schools have seen their capacities diminish significantly due to the effects of AIDS (poverty, disease and hunger) and are no longer able to participate in self-help activities in the schools.

– However, the educational system also has great potential in the fight against AIDS:

> The educational sector has an important role to play in the fight against AIDS through the inclusion of HIV/AIDS in curricula. Children who do not attend school must be reached through the informal educational sector.

- The integration of education on sexuality and HIV/AIDS into curricula and the development of anti-AIDS clubs or similar groups can raise AIDS awareness and provide students with life skills that help them to protect themselves and others against infection.
- Education on human rights and HIV can reduce stigma and contribute to greater openness about HIV.

– HIV prevention should be conducted in formal and informal segments of the educational system. Informal components can include peer education, youth groups, church groups and so on.

– In the initial years of the HIV epidemic there was identified a partially positive correlation between school education and HIV infection: the risk of having multiple sexual partners and being infected with HIV increased with the level of education. This connection was linked to the greater mobility and the more "liberal" values of the better-educated and high-income groups. In recent years, however, these correlations appear to have reversed. Data from Zambia indicate that, in the cities, the HIV prevalence among young people with moderate and high levels of edu-

---

Best Practice

UNICEF: My future is my choice

The "My future is my choice Life Skills Programme" in Windhoek, Namibia, has been jointly conducted by the Namibian government and UNICEF since 1997. Its objective is, through sex education, to strengthen the communication, negotiation and decision-making skills of young people, so that they can safeguard their sexual health and protect themselves against HIV infection. More than 50,000 young people have participated in Life Skills Training, educational and informational materials have been distributed, and the private sector and NGOs are actively involved in the programme. Significant obstacles to implementation are the continuing financial bottlenecks and sustaining the interest of volunteers. The programme has succeeded in reducing the risk behaviour of young people. It was important to create an enabling environment which made behaviour change possible. The participation of young people themselves is the primary factor in the success of the programme: they help in the planning, conduct (as peer educators) the Life Skills Training and its supervision and are engaged in operational research. Young people are successful as peer educators because they can discuss sensitive areas of sexuality. They have the necessary interest and the energy to work as peer educators; however, it is necessary to develop their skills for doing so (UNICEF).

cation is falling, while among young people with a low level of education it is rising. This observation suggests that the effect of education is now to reduce susceptibility to HIV. The observed increase in the HIV prevalence among young people with a low level of education is very disturbing, and calls for urgent action (Kelly 1999; Fylkesnes 2001).

7.5 HEALTH SECTOR

- In many of the most heavily affected countries, health systems lack adequate resources and cannot offer appropriate, affordable and high-quality care to their population. HIV/AIDS puts additional pressure on the health systems through:
  - An increasing number of AIDS patients.
  - Displacement of patients with other illnesses.
  - Increase of tuberculosis patients due to the mutually reinforcing HIV and tuberculosis epidemics.
  - Chronic illness and death of health workers. In several countries health facilities are losing a large percentage of their employees.

> AIDS is straining healthcare systems through increasing the numbers of HIV/AIDS patients and the loss of health workers.

- Studies in Botswana, for example, have shown that in several hospitals up to 80 per cent of the adult patients and around 30 per cent of the children have HIV-related diseases. Employees complain of burn-out, since the time demanded for diagnoses and examinations has increased by 30 per cent, the demand for counselling has risen, and the care of the growing number of dying patients creates psychological problems. Staff shortages are becoming a problem in public hospitals, since many health workers are either switching to private clinics or emigrating. The government in Botswana fears that HIV/AIDS will overwhelm the healthcare system if no adequate interventions are undertaken (Botswana 2000).
- In many developing countries, church health facilities provide a substantial proportion of healthcare. Their contribution and potential in the fight against HIV/AIDS should therefore not be underestimated, especially in times of worsening government healthcare.

8. Stigma and discrimination

8.1 HIV-ASSOCIATED STIGMA AND DISCRIMINATION

> HIV is associated with stigma and discrimination which constitute a fundamental obstacle in the fight against HIV/AIDS.

- Almost everywhere, HIV/AIDS remains associated with stigma and discrimination. Stigma and rejection lead to individual suffering for the persons against whom they are applied. They constitute a fundamental obstacle in the fight against HIV/AIDS, since they make open discussion more difficult.

- Stigmatization often leads to discrimination, where people are unjustly treated and disadvantaged on the basis of their HIV infection, or due to them being affected by HIV (e.g. as orphans and widows). People living with HIV/AIDS (PLWHA) are often exposed to complex forms of discrimination, and are discriminated against not only because of their HIV status (e.g. women who are HIV-positive).

- Prejudices against PLWHA normally derive from already existing fears and prejudices about women, sexuality, poverty, and so on. AIDS is often regarded as an illness which men get from prostitutes or as a consequence of promiscuity. Among women it is seen to be caused by prostitution, sex outside of marriage or with multiple partners. Sometimes HIV is also seen as a woman's disease, like other sexually transmitted illnesses. Women are then accused of transmitting HIV and being responsible for spreading it (UNAIDS/WHO 2001).

> PLWHA frequently experience rejection and exclusion in families, communities and at the workplace.

- Often, HIV-positive people experience rejection and exclusion in families and communities, through refusal of care, loss of living space, neglect, physical violence, and the collapse of partnerships and marriages.

- For example, in Uganda in the early 1990s, community members refused to care for HIV-infected persons, as they were fearful of becoming infected themselves or they feared the related costs. Many people blamed others for the epidemic. This resulted in people not assuming responsibility for the epidemic, but rather regarding it as a problem for others. To combat the HIV epidemic successfully, however, it was essential to reduce stigma and discrimination (UNAIDS 2001b).

- The International Labour Organization (ILO) has stated in its Code of Practice that for successful HIV prevention in the workplace it is necessary that HIV/AIDS be treated like any other illness, that working people may not be discriminated against or stigmatized on the basis of their HIV status, and that HIV tests cannot be made a requirement for hiring or remaining employed (ILO 2001).

- However, discrimination is by no means universal. There are very many examples in which people who are HIV-infected and those who are affected by HIV are accepted by their partners and families and integrated into their communities.

8.2 Denial

- Stigmatization and the taboo of HIV/AIDS mean that people repress the subject of HIV and thus avoid dealing with it. On the individual level, denial means not wanting to admit to infection, or the possibility of infection. An individual may not acknowledge that they have to deal with the threat and may have to change intimate behaviour, probably for the rest of their life, and under certain circumstances against significant resistances from outside. Denial is also promoted by the fact that many people in poor countries see the diagnosis of HIV as tantamount to a death sentence, since virtually no treatment has been available in the absence of antiretroviral therapy programmes. On the community and national levels, denial of HIV means that important and controversial themes in the fight against HIV – such as cultural standards of sexuality and inequalities in gender relations and social life – are evaded.

> Stigmatization and the taboo of HIV/AIDS cause people to shun the subject of HIV and repress it. Such denial in turn leads to stigmatization.

- Denial in turn promotes stigmatization and discrimination. People resist dealing with unpleasant and frightening themes, and they discriminate against others who do actively confront such issues. Denial leads to silence about HIV, which becomes a fundamental obstacle in fighting HIV/AIDS.
- Here, however, the HIV epidemic also offers an opportunity. Overcoming denial opens up possibilities for addressing social inequalities and taboo themes (e.g. sexual violence) and achieving social renewal.

8.3 Sexuality and taboo

- Silence also frequently shrouds the themes of sexuality and death, which are intimately related to HIV. They fall under a certain taboo in almost every society and cannot, at least in public discussions, be named and addressed easily. In most societies risks were associated with sexual intercourse, such as sexually transmitted infections and unwanted pregnancies. However, these are generally not mortal threats.
- Moreover, HIV casts a deep shadow over sexuality, since sexual intercourse, which actually creates life, is associated with the risk of death.
- In fighting AIDS one should not convey negative messages about sexuality. Such messages lack credibility and do long-term harm, even if they might initially appear to promise results.
- The churches, too, must critically analyse their messages about sexuality in many areas. Sexuality should be presented as a gift from God with which people must deal responsibly. Such a change of consciousness will then also have a beneficial influence in other areas (e.g. the self-determination of women).

> AIDS education should not convey negative messages about sexuality. The objective is to deal with sexuality responsibly and understand it as a gift from God.

8.4 Overcoming stigma

- Breaking through the cycle of stigma–rejection–denial is of fundamental importance in the fight against HIV. "Breaking the silence" has become a central concept in many discussions and programmes. Adequate strategies must be adapted to the specific context. The

> Breaking the silence about HIV and overcoming stigma can occur through inclusion of people living with HIV and care for people affected by HIV (including antiretroviral treatment).

following interventions have been shown to be effective in overcoming stigma:

- The inclusion and active participation of people living with HIV/AIDS is absolutely necessary.
- The creation of possibilities and options for PLWHA, such as support groups and self-help groups, an informed and balanced diet, changing habits which have a negative impact (e.g. alcohol consumption) and generally a positive attitude, that is positive living, decrease denial and stigma.
- Providing care for PLWHA contributes to destigmatizing HIV/AIDS. This communicates the message that something very concrete can be done for HIV-infected people. The predominant question for HIV-infected people is often what will happen with their children if they die. Structures working in partnership to care for orphans are often very helpful in this case.
- Access to antiretroviral drugs is of great significance. It has been shown that through increased access to life-prolonging ARV therapy and the hope this brings, more people will be open about their HIV infection, will go for HIV testing, and AIDS will become a "normal" disease.
- Openly addressing the subject of HIV – in all possible places and occasions – contributes to removing the taboo.
- One should entirely avoid concepts such as "AIDS victims", since they contribute to further stigmatization and disempower PLWHA.

> Churches have recognized that they have often contributed to stigmatization and silence. One of their main tasks is to fight the stigma and accept PLWHA.

– Churches have an important role to play in all of these areas. In Africa, the churches have increasingly made efforts to break the silence about AIDS and to combat stigma and discrimination within communities. At the Ecumenical Consultation on HIV/AIDS of the churches in Nairobi in November 2001, stigma was identified as the main theme in the fight against AIDS. The churches were called upon to fight stigma and discrimination and no longer exclude HIV-positive people, but rather to accept them (Ecumenical Consultation 2001). Churches have increasingly addressed stigma as their main contribution in the fight against HIV/AIDS.

8.5 Demystifying HIV/AIDS

– In people's minds, HIV is often primarily associated with Africa. It coincides with an image of Africa which is largely characterized by wars, catastrophes and hopelessness. These images should be contradicted and the disease should be demystified.

– HIV is an illness which can be transmitted sexually, through shared use of injection equipment, through blood transfusions and from mother to child, as is the case with several other diseases. For example, hepatitis B has similar transmission routes, but it has not the same symbolic charge as AIDS.

– The moral and ethical aspects of HIV, such as extramarital sexual intercourse, are important questions in their own right. However, there are good reasons for not mixing them up from the start with the fight against HIV: HIV infection is *not* caused by having multiple sexual partners, but rather through the transmission of a virus from one person to another. It is the *risk* of infection that is increased through multiple partners and unprotected sexual intercourse. Moreover, the risk is substantially dependent on the HIV prevalence in a given context.

- People are infected with HIV or affected by HIV, but there are no grounds here to ask about "guilt" or to condemn certain behaviour.

- In general, those affected by HIV infection are attributed a far greater burden of guilt for the infection/illness than is the case for other diseases, such as malaria. One normally does not condemn people for having failed to sleep under a mosquito net and therefore contracting malaria. In the latter case, one proceeds to investigate the social and psychological conditions of mosquito net usage, and not to stigmatize those who fall sick with malaria for their disease (Byamugisha 2000).

- The equation of immoral behaviour in sexual matters with HIV infection can lead to the infection and illness being regarded as a punishment from God for misbehaviour. This increases stigmatization, excludes those affected from the religious community, and can subjectively bar access to God's healing power.

> HIV infection is frequently accompanied by an attribution of guilt to the affected persons, as a consequence of which people can be banished from the religious community. Moral aspects of sexual behaviour are on a different level, however, and should not be mixed up with the discussion about HIV as illness.

9. Human rights

9.1 HUMAN RIGHTS FRAMEWORK

> HIV and human rights are interconnected in various ways. Human rights violations increase vulnerability to HIV infection.

- Since the foundation of the United Nations, human rights instruments have been developed which have attained universal recognition: the Universal Declaration of Human Rights, the Covenant on Economic, Social and Cultural Rights and the Covenant on Civil and Political Rights. These laws define human rights and establish, for the states which have ratified the pacts, internationally binding standards for their protection and promotion (United Nations 1966a, 1966b).

- Human rights are universal (they apply for every person, always and everywhere), inalienable (one cannot take away or give away a right), and indivisible (there are no hierarchies of rights).

- HIV and human rights are connected with one another in various ways, and the human rights of those affected by HIV can be violated. Human rights violations increase vulnerability and infection risk. Global obligations entail a responsibility to protect and promote human rights.

- The Ecumenical Advocacy Alliance (2001b) states that the human dignity of people living with HIV/AIDS is best safeguarded by protecting their human rights and by promoting an attitude of concern for and solidarity with them.

- The UN Commission on Human Rights, referring to human rights laws, declared in its resolutions that discrimination against a person on the basis of that person's health status – including HIV/AIDS – is inadmissible (UN Commission on Human Rights 1999, 2001). Therefore, discrimination against people living with HIV is a violation of their human rights.

> The right to adequate treatment for HIV is part of the fundamental human right to health.

- The right to health and the right to life are fundamental human rights which are defined in the human rights instruments. These rights are violated by the lack of access of HIV-infected persons to adequate care and treatment, including treatment of opportunistic diseases and treatment with life-prolonging antiretroviral drugs.

- The Commission on Human Rights of the UN has repeatedly defined the right to adequate therapy for AIDS as part of the right to health (UN Commission on Human Rights 2001).

- The description of the population groups with high HIV risk makes clear that it primarily involves groups suffering from human rights violations. CSWs, men who have sex with men, injecting drug users, refugees, migrants, etc. are often discriminated against, sometimes criminalized, often exposed to government and private violence, have less access to healthcare and, on the whole, have fewer options for shaping their own lives. They are therefore exposed to the risk of HIV infection without being able to influence this situation directly.

9.2 International obligations in the human rights context

- It is generally recognized that individual states have obligations to protect and promote human rights within their national borders. However, international human rights laws also define obligations of states to cooperate internationally with respect to realizing human rights on the international scale. Accordingly, states also have a duty to promote, respect and protect human rights vis-à-vis populations of other countries.

> States also have a duty vis-à-vis the populations of other countries to promote, respect and protect human rights. They are therefore obliged, via their policies, not to promote HIV transmission in other countries.

- In the context of HIV, such a claim leads to an obligation on the rich countries to make it possible for the poor countries to fight AIDS adequately. This can be done by increasing development aid and shaping international trade agreements to increase the resources of poor countries. From a rigorous application of human rights laws it follows that access to antiretroviral drugs is a human right within the framework of the right to health. Under the obligation of states to cooperate, rich countries must guarantee access to adequate antiretroviral treatment via measures such as application of the patent laws of the WTO in accordance with human rights principles (Weinreich 2002).

- UN organizations are increasingly recognizing the global obligations of the states in this connection. An essential provision of their guidelines on HIV/AIDS and human rights was revised in August 2002. Under the new provision, access to antiretroviral treatment is a right which states must guarantee through cooperation (OHCHR/UNAIDS 2002).

9.3 Public health and human rights

- Many goals and strategies in the fight against AIDS must be established in a longer-term perspective. They are aimed at improving the living conditions of the poor and disadvantaged, preserving their dignity and implementing human rights within the universal framework, through fundamental social changes such as reduction of poverty, changes in gender relations, enhancing food security, striving for peace in war and conflict zones, and exerting influence on rich countries and international financial institutions to provide greater support and eliminate the disadvantaging of poor countries.

> To fight AIDS effectively, the socio-economic context and the gender relations which promote vulnerability to HIV infection must be changed.

- In order to counter HIV/AIDS effectively, strategies and goals are also necessary which contribute to lowering HIV transmission in the shorter term. However, short- and long-term goals and strategies are not rigidly distinct from one another, and must not be placed in opposition. Two examples:

  - A short-term objective such as increased utilization of HIV tests cannot be attained through measures which run contrary to the fundamental and long-term goal of promoting human rights. Therefore, compulsory HIV testing, for example, is not an effective strategy in HIV prevention.

  - The lowering of HIV prevalence among CSWs cannot be attained through programmes which criminalize prostitution, put pressure on affected women and violate their human rights.

> Short- and long-term strategies must not be seen in opposition to one another: e.g. HIV must not be combated at the expense of human rights.

– Studies and observations have shown that, besides the violation of human rights which is expressed in such programmes, these interventions are also not effective from the public health and epidemiological point of view in the fight against HIV.

10. People living with HIV/AIDS (PLWHA)

- The concept of positive living counters the hopelessness associated for many people with HIV, by emphasizing that a positive life with an HIV infection is possible. The concept of "people living with HIV/AIDS" (PLWHA) is meant to express life with HIV, and that HIV infection is not synonymous with dying and death, even in the absence of antiretroviral therapy. Such a concept should not play down the fact that a life with HIV is in fact often difficult. However, even under conditions of poverty, the attitude towards one's own infection and disease is essential. The term "AIDS victim" helps disempower people living with HIV.

  > The concept of "people living with HIV/AIDS" should make clear that it is about living with HIV, not dying of it. The term "AIDS victim" helps disempower people living with HIV.

- Negative messages on posters and in the media which emphasize that "AIDS kills" contribute to further denial of HIV. For example, in Uganda, which is seen as an example of a successful fight against the spread of HIV/AIDS, it was recognized that instilling fear about AIDS is counter-productive and should be replaced by positive messages which give people hope (Okware et al. 2001).

  > Fear-inducing messages are counter-productive in the fight against AIDS, since they increase stigma and denial.

- There are no "guilty" and "innocent" "AIDS victims". No illness may be regarded as a punishment for behaviour. As is well known, people who smoke have a much higher risk of dying of lung cancer than non-smokers. Nevertheless, lung cancer is not regarded as a punishment for smoking, but rather as a consequence, which moreover does not necessarily occur, but rather only with a certain likelihood. It would be ethically incorrect for doctors and family members to refuse aid on the theory that the patient was to blame for developing the disease.

  > AIDS is not a punishment for past behaviour, but rather an illness which occurs with a certain probability (given a certain behaviour).

- One must clearly distinguish between the illness and the patient, and between the infection and those who are affected. One must convey the message that HIV infection is to be avoided, because it may lead to disease and death, but that nevertheless there is a positive life with HIV, and therefore one should have the courage to address the topic of HIV openly.

- The human dignity of HIV-infected persons must be respected and protected. The Ecumenical Advocacy Alliance (2001) says that the starting point of every action must be recognition and respect for the dignity of the individual, irrespective of the situation, because Christians believe that human beings are formed in God's image.

- In the fight against HIV/AIDS, PLWHA are important resource persons. If they are ready to speak openly about their HIV infection, they can contribute decisively to prevention efforts by making a personal impact on listeners and giving HIV a human face.

- However, it is a major challenge and strain for HIV-infected people to tell their own story over and over, to share information on intimate matters, and thereby in part to experience stigma and rejection.

- Many HIV-positive people find it liberating to deal openly with their own infection and moreover are motivated by a desire to protect other people from HIV infection and to give hope to those already infected.

  > HIV-positive people who deal openly with their infection can make a personal impact and are credible witnesses.

- The more people admit to their HIV status, the simpler it will be for those who come later. Groups of people living openly with their HIV infection can be formed on the community level, within the framework of HIV testing centres, and on the national level in networks. Well-known personalities who are recognized and active in public life and who live openly with HIV can serve as identification figures and role models.

11. Prevention

11.1 SIGNIFICANCE OF PREVENTION

- The prevention of HIV infections is of great significance, since this avoids disease, premature death and the social impact of the HIV epidemic. The importance of prevention is further emphasized by the fact that there is no cure for the infection, and, although there has been some progress on access to ARV therapy, the possibilities for treatment in poor countries are still limited.
- According to estimates, of the 45 million new HIV infections expected worldwide by the year 2010, 29 million could be stopped by adequate prevention measures. The prerequisite for this would be the adequate provision of resources (Stover et al. 2002).
- It always pays to invest early in prevention. Ultimately, these expenditures are more than offset by savings on follow-up costs imposed on society when the epidemic spreads. Prevention in an area with a generally lower HIV prevalence (such as in Asia and Latin America) can however represent a greater challenge, since the social consequences of the illness are not (yet) visible there on a larger scale.
- It cannot be overemphasized, however, that one cannot simply trust that a low HIV prevalence in one country or one population group will always remain low. That everything possible must be done early on in order to prevent an increase in infections is an important lesson which should be drawn from the epidemic, which has existed for 20 years now. Decision-makers in the affected countries, churches, ecumenical partners and everyone who has access to the corresponding information and resources have a special responsibility here.

> It is always worthwhile for states and communities to invest early in prevention, since it avoids the high follow-up costs of a growing HIV epidemic. Churches and ecumenical partners have a special responsibility here.

11.2 EFFECTIVE PREVENTION

- Various prevention strategies have proven to be effective: voluntary counselling and testing (Sweat et al. 2000), condom use (Lagarde et al. 2001), reduction in the number of sexual partners and raising of the age of first sexual activity (UNAIDS 2002). The following have been identified as determinants of successful HIV prevention (UNAIDS 2000):
  - a political context which actively supports prevention;
  - the active role of communities and grassroots initiatives;
  - involvement of people living with HIV;
  - communication and information, including education on sexual and reproductive health;
  - creation of an enabling environment which puts people in a position to protect themselves and others from infection;
  - integrating role models and outstanding personalities in the fight against AIDS;
  - combating and reducing stigma, discrimination, denial and taboos;
  - breaking the silence surrounding HIV;

> Effective prevention interventions are: voluntary counselling and testing; condom use; reduction in the number of sexual partners; combating stigma; promotion of human rights.

- protecting and promoting human rights, including the rights of women and children;
- treating sexually transmitted infections;
- integrating prevention, care and mitigation of the impact of HIV/AIDS;
- increased access to ARV therapy.

> Active participation of the (affected) communities is the central element in successful AIDS interventions.

— It has been demonstrated that the active participation of communities is the central element in successful AIDS interventions. This requires the elimination of stigma, partnerships between non-governmental organizations and governmental organizations, and the systematic inclusion of people and groups living with HIV.

Best Practice

Ministry of Health/German Technical Cooperation (GTZ) AIDS Control Project Mbeya

The Mbeya region in Tanzania has a population of 2 million people, most of whom are farmers. In several sub-areas of the region, the HIV prevalence has reached 30 per cent. This makes the Mbeya the hardest-hit region in Tanzania, after Dar es Salaam. The Mbeya Regional AIDS Control Programme integrates all aspects of HIV/AIDS and STI control in a single programme. The programme is implemented through the existing structures of the health sector. Since 1988 GTZ has supported the Tanzanian Health Ministry in implementing the programme by providing up to 90 per cent of the funds for HIV/AIDS work. The churches, which provide a large share of the healthcare in the region, are involved as an essential partner. The achievements of the programme include the following: the rate of HIV infections among pregnant women fell from 20 per cent in 1994 to 15 per cent in 1999; an estimated 60 per cent of all AIDS patients receive home care; most of the health facilities offer treatment for STIs; and the district councils and communities have begun to finance some of the programmes themselves. Essential to this success has been the fact that, from the start of the programme, GTZ's commitment was planned for more than 10 years, so that there was enough time to develop and test interventions and to demonstrate results. Beyond this, GTZ is pursuing a participatory approach and promotes capacity building on all levels (Ministry of Health Tanzania/GTZ 2000).

— The spread of HIV is not determined by any one single factor. While sexual behaviour is frequently the most important factor influencing dissemination, this behaviour varies very widely between cultures, age groups, socio-economic status and gender.
— Sexual behaviour itself is determined by a range of factors. For example, it has been shown that a greater number of sexual partners is associated with a greater probability of HIV infection. The chances of individuals having intercourse with CSWs and thereby having more partners are higher when large numbers of male labour migrants live together.

These communities, however, develop through a complex interplay of economic and historical factors: mineworkers in southern Africa, forced migration due to war, long journeys on transit routes, and the lack of a secure livelihood are some of the factors.

- An epidemiological study published in 2001 investigated the conditions of HIV dissemination in four African cities, two of which have a high HIV prevalence: Kisumu, Kenya, and Ndola, Zambia; and two with lower HIV prevalence: Yaoundé, Cameroon, and Cotonou, Benin (Buvé et al. 2001). The most widespread biological and behavioural factors in the high-prevalence cities were: low age of women at time of first sexual intercourse, low age at time of first marriage, age difference between husband and wife, the presence of herpes simplex-2-infection and trichomoniasis (both STIs), and absence of circumcision among men.

- Added to this is the fact that a large share of the African population is very young and therefore has a higher probability of being sexually active. This also contributes to the relatively higher incidence of HIV and other STIs in Africa.

- When these factors are not present, the epidemic can remain hidden for many years. In the presence of the biological, social and economic factors which promote dissemination, the epidemic can expand rapidly.

- One frequently hears the argument that the HIV epidemic has been around for more than 20 years and is by now well known to people, yet little has changed. This is contradicted in a number of ways which make the slow response of many countries and societies more understandable:

    - As the examples above demonstrate, there are indeed solid indications of the effectiveness of prevention.
    - It should not be forgotten that, in the initial years, the HIV epidemic only appeared in isolated areas, and thus was not highly visible. An understanding of a global epidemic (pandemic) has only developed in the last 10 years.
    - In contrast to people working in this field in the rich countries, the global epidemiological data on HIV/AIDS are not available for many people in poor countries. Even if epidemiological data were to be available, it would be difficult to integrate them into the reality of people's lives.
    - People living under conditions of poverty and deprivation often lack options to change their own lives in such a way that they could adequately deal with AIDS. They are exposed to structural relations over which they have little individual influence, but which at the same time make them highly vulnerable to HIV infection. Under these circumstances, an adequate response to HIV through behaviour change, which is often simply seen as related to sexual behaviour, in isolation of the social context is frequently impossible.

> When enhancing factors are not present, the epidemic can remain hidden for many years. In the presence of the biological, social and economic factors which promote dissemination, the epidemic can expand rapidly.

11.3 Prevention programmes

- HIV prevention must be embedded in the social context of the people. This applies both to prevention targeted at groups especially exposed to a risk, and the general population (Piot and Coll-Seck 2001).
- In the fight against HIV, often too many simplistic and authoritarian models have been followed, instead of trying more holistic interventions. For example, thus far sexual behaviour has not been looked at sufficiently in its social context.
- The scope and extent of existing prevention programmes are often inadequate: prevention has not yet (or not yet adequately) reached many people (e.g. children and young people who do not attend school) (UNICEF/UNAIDS/WHO 2002). Prevention campaigns which utilize the written word fail to reach many segments of the rural population (in Ethiopia, for example, 75 per cent of all women are illiterate).
- The message of behaviour change – or in the case of a non-risk behaviour, behaviour reinforcement – requires repetition and amplification in order to reach people. A one-time campaign is not enough.
- Moreover, different methods (peer education, mass campaigns, counselling, etc.) complement one another and must not be seen as mutually exclusive.
- Affected people must be actively included in the planning and implementation of interventions. Only in this way can sustainability be attained. In addition, active involvement with the material generates an awareness and learning effect.
- HIV/AIDS is intimately connected with taboo themes: sexuality, dying and death. In individuals and within communities these are frequently linked with fears and barriers. Simple communication of knowledge (e.g. of the medical facts) can have only a limited effect. Such communication has its place, but it must be supplemented by other methods (e.g. through the testimony of people living with HIV).
- Education must take place cautiously and deal with people's foreknowledge, fears and current situation. Disadvantaged and marginalized groups must be supported in their efforts to implement educational content:
    - Explaining the significance of condoms for preventing HIV infection to a woman living in a South African village is unlikely to have much impact if she cannot overcome corresponding obstacles: under some circumstances there simply may be no condoms available in her area, she may have no money to buy them, she may lack the confidence to buy them, she might not be able to speak with her partner about their use for fear of stigmatization, and her partner will probably refuse to use them anyway.
    - Explaining the significance of premarital abstinence for HIV prevention to a young man in a poor area in Nairobi cannot be very effective if he hears from his friends that unprotected sexual intercourse is something fundamental to being a man, when he has no future prospects and does not know whether he will ever be able to marry and sustain a family, and when no one else around him ever speaks openly about responsible sexual behaviour.

> The scope and extent of existing prevention programmes are often inadequate. Young people in particular are often not reached.

> Affected people and communities must actively participate in the planning and implementation of interventions.

- Prevention must also address human rights, discrimination and stigma. When people fear stigmatization in their family or community, it is less likely that they will look for or accept prevention information. In the same way, access to ARV therapy increases and supports prevention interventions.
- Networking of programmes and initiatives is important to avoid them from acting in isolation, to deploy limited resources efficiently, to avoid duplication, and to achieve the greatest possible integration into communities.
- In many countries, successful HIV/AIDS interventions already exist in various areas. However, until now, most programmes have only been implemented on a small scale (regionally, related to a certain group, etc.). Scaling up (full-scale introduction) of successful interventions is an urgent necessity.
- Along with this, however, further research is also necessary, since in many cases the best method is not known (Global HIV Prevention Working Group 2002).
- However, examples of successful interventions cannot always be simply transposed from one country to another, because the respective specific situations must be considered.

> It is urgently necessary to scale up successful interventions. Besides this, however, further research is also necessary, since in many cases the best measures are still not known.

11.4 INFORMATION, EDUCATION AND COMMUNICATION

- Information, education and communication (IEC) are indispensable for conveying to people knowledge about AIDS. In countries where prevention has been successfully implemented, an education component generally forms an essential part of their interventions.
- Preventive education campaigns should reach everyone, including those who are hard to reach, such as young people, women and minorities. In many population groups there still exists a shortage of information about HIV/AIDS and how one can protect oneself against it. Studies have shown that even in countries with high HIV prevalence, a substantial proportion of young girls are not acting on the assumption that they run a risk of HIV infection.
- Appropriate messages must also be conveyed to succeeding generations.
- A representative study in South Africa found that the main contents of HIV/AIDS education were generally well understood. The vast majority of those surveyed, however, indicated that they needed further information about the disease, sexual abuse, condom use and negotiations, etc. (HSRC 2002).
- Moreover, experiences from churches and community-based organizations demonstrate that in general there is still a lack of adequate knowledge about HIV/AIDS, especially among the poor and people living in rural areas.
- HIV information campaigns should involve NGOs and community groups. The churches have an invaluable potential here, thanks to their infrastructure and networks, which reach into the most remote areas.

> Information, education and communication are indispensable in the fight against AIDS. One must also ensure that appropriate messages are conveyed to succeeding generations of young people.

- Messages about HIV and sexuality are generally more readily accepted when they come from a member of one's own group (e.g. among school children when they come from classmates). Trust is greater here, because such a person comes from the same situation and thus understands one's own problems.

- Such so-called peer education has proven to be effective among school children, CSWs, students, the rural population and others. The change can take place on the individual level of the affected persons, but also on the level of communities and groups. The latter are encouraged to undertake common actions which result in changes of policies and programmes. For peer education programmes to succeed it is necessary that peer educators be carefully selected, receive specific training, and that their motivation be maintained and promoted (UNAIDS 1999).

- As with all interventions in the fight against HIV/AIDS, HIV education should not be exclusively focused on HIV. In order to integrate the discussion about HIV into people's everyday lives, HIV/AIDS must be dealt with in the overall context of sexual health, gender role behaviour, etc.

- Another effective method employs drama and role plays, in which situations from everyday life are played out, often in an improvised manner, thereby creating awareness and concern. Opportunities to role play can be found in many groups, and they are already being conducted in many places, above all by youth groups, post-test clubs, home care groups, etc. Drama and role plays should not be used as an isolated strategy, since their influence on behaviour change on the whole is limited.

- "Outreach" means that instruction and education are implemented, proceeding from centres. Thus, people living with HIV can report about their own experiences in communities, church groups, schools, etc. This can be done together with peer educators, with the professional staff from counselling centres, and so on.

11.5 Voluntary Counselling and Testing (VCT)

11.5.1 Preventive effect

- 95 per cent of people in poor countries – including HIV-infected persons – have no knowledge of their own HIV status. There are several reasons for this:
  - HIV testing and counselling services are not available in sufficient quantity.
  - Tests are often relatively expensive compared to people's incomes. Many people, above all in rural areas, have little or no money, since they live from subsistence agriculture.
  - The demand for HIV tests is often low because of predominant stigma and lack of treatment, which make many people fearful of a positive HIV test result.

- VCT has a preventive effect on HIV transmission. A large-scale study in Kenya, Tanzania and Trinidad found that HIV-positive men and women who received VCT had significantly less unprotected sexual

intercourse with their partners than those who received only health education (Voluntary HIV-1 Counselling and Testing Efficacy Group 2000).
– VCT is a cost-effective prevention intervention. Model calculations for Kenya and Tanzania conclude that it costs 249 or 346 US dollars to prevent an HIV infection via VCT (Sweat et al. 2000). Offering more VCT is therefore a necessary HIV prevention measure.
– Despite many efforts to promote VCT, the uptake has in many settings been low. Demand for VCT has however usually increased considerably once ARV therapy has been offered to people who test HIV+ve, as is shown by the experience of ARV pilot programmes.

11.5.2 VCT programmes

– HIV testing without adequate counselling is not helpful, but rather in many cases can be harmful. Counselling before the test (pre-test counselling) should prepare people for a positive test result. In addition, support must be on hand after the test, since many clients experience a positive test result as a shock. The counselling allows people to recognize problems, devise solution strategies and finally gives support in coping with the consequences of HIV. Clients should also have the possibility and be encouraged to come to further counselling sessions (follow-up counselling). Experience in existing programmes shows that many clients accept the offer, and the counsellor becomes an important contact person for clients in dealing with their HIV problems.

> HIV tests without appropriate counselling are not helpful, but rather in many cases can be harmful. Compulsory testing is unethical and does not serve the purpose of HIV prevention.

– If someone tests HIV negative, receiving confirmation of their own negative HIV status can constitute a major incentive for making a behaviour change, or for retaining the sexual behaviour which preserves this negative HIV status. Counselling of HIV-negative clients is of great importance, since one must make sure that people who have received a negative HIV test result do not mistakenly conclude that they are "not susceptible to HIV", and then expose themselves to the risk of HIV transmission.

> Knowledge of one's own negative HIV status can constitute a major incentive to preserve HIV negative status. Special weight is given to the HIV tests of HIV-negative people. HIV tests must be affordable for the poor.

– All measures which rely on an element of force, such as compulsory tests, compulsory reporting of HIV status or obligatory provision of names of HIV-positive clients to the supervisory authorities, are not only unethical, but also do nothing to help fight HIV, since they promote denial and stigmatization (UNAIDS 2000a).

– Not only people active in the field of medicine should be trained as counsellors, but also community workers, clergy, volunteers in home care projects, etc. The skills which are learned for counselling facilitate more generally access to HIV awareness and allow people to talk about HIV.

> As counsellors, one should train not only people who are active in the medical field, but also clergy, home care staff, community workers and so on.

– In the medical field there is sometimes a tendency to place priority in VCT on HIV testing of patients. Under conditions of scarce resources, however, this does not appear justified, when the test result cannot affect the therapy decision.

– When testing patients one must at least provide counselling and education, so that the patient actually benefits from the test, or at least is not harmed by it. Furthermore, one must take care that a positive test result does not lead to discrimination against patients, or even a refusal of treatment.

- Clients receive mutual support in self-help groups, which can be affiliated to a counselling centre. They create an environment in which people are enabled to live with their HIV illness.
- HIV testing must be affordable for the poor. Even a "nominal" financial charge can dissuade poor people from HIV testing.

11.5.3 Disclosure of test results

> Counselling should enable people to disclose their HIV status to others, and above all to their sexual partners.

- Disclosure of HIV status, above all to sexual partner(s), is important for effective prevention. However, many people refuse to tell anyone about their HIV test result. In a study conducted in Dar es Salaam, women listed the greatest obstacles that prevented them from taking an HIV test and communicating the test results: fear of their partner's reaction; decision-making power and communication structures between the partners; and a negative attitude of the partner toward HIV tests (Maman et al. 2001). The objective of counselling must therefore be to enable people to communicate their HIV status (positive or negative) to others.
- In principle, VCT strives to advise marriage and sexual partners together, in order to guarantee that the partners know each other's HIV status. Problems can develop here, however, because of the unequal distribution of power in many partner relationships. Communication of a positive test result sometimes gives rise to violence or to the break-up of the relationship. The weaker partner – often, but not always, the female – must be protected. Thus, neither of the partners should be pressured into agreeing to an HIV test.
- A cornerstone of VCT is the confidentiality (similar to that between doctor and patient) which exists between counsellor and client: test results, and even the fact that an HIV test was performed, may not be passed on to others, and all contents of the counselling must remain confidential.

11.5.4 Pre-marital testing

> In principle, HIV tests before a planned marriage should be viewed positively. Churches should not, however, make a negative HIV test for both partners a condition for performing a marriage.

- In general, HIV tests for partners before a marriage should be seen as something positive. They are a means to foster awareness of HIV and to counsel the partners. However, they should be performed as early as possible before a planned marriage, in order to spare the partners from being confronted with almost insoluble psychological difficulties.
- Some churches make a negative HIV test for both partners a condition for a church wedding. This practice is questionable for two reasons:
  - It is by no means certain that, after the refusal of marriage by the church, the affected partner(s) will not infect others with HIV.
  - Marriage rests on the affection and love of the partners. This remains valid even when one partner is HIV-positive.
- If partners so wish, therefore, it should be possible for them to marry even in the event of a positive test result for one or both of them. A prerequisite, of course, is that both partners should be completely informed about their respective HIV statuses.
- To disclose HIV test results to others than the partners is incompatible with the confidentiality of such information, which derives from the protection of the individual's privacy, and moreover generally results in a

stigmatization of those who are affected. Third persons should not learn of the test results without the consent of those tested.

11.6 CONDOMS

11.6.1 Male condoms

- The use of latex condoms to prevent the exchange of body fluids during sexual intercourse is an essential element of all HIV prevention efforts. The strategy of safer sex essentially rests on the regular and proper use of condoms.
- In many countries, especially in North America and Europe, HIV transmission rates have been reduced with the aid of widespread campaigns promoting the use of condoms. In Thailand, too, a large-scale action to promote the use of condoms made an essential contribution to reducing HIV/AIDS.
- Several problem areas have to be distinguished here. First of all, the question arises as to the scientific facts about the effectiveness of using condoms to prevent HIV transmission. The most comprehensive study on the matter was published in 2001. After examining all of the published data, an experts' workshop came to the following conclusions (NIAID/NIH/DHHS 2001):
  - Regular and correct use of latex condoms can exclude the transmission of HIV between an infected and an uninfected sexual partner with almost 100 per cent certainty. The argument that condoms often contain pores which are larger than the virus itself is inconclusive, since it is exclusively the exchange of fluid which is decisive, and this is almost entirely prevented.
  - In reality, however, one cannot proceed on the assumption that a condom is always used correctly, that condoms always possess a constant quality, etc. Therefore, effective protection is not 100 per cent, but 85 per cent. This means that couples where one partner is HIV-infected and condoms are always used run a risk of infecting the other partner with HIV 85 per cent below that of couples who never use condoms.
- In many countries, however, there are religious and cultural reservations about promoting the use of condoms. Often, churches argue that encouraging condom use will increase and condone promiscuity. They argue that this is morally unacceptable and also does not contribute to containing the HIV epidemic. There are no empirical studies, however, which support this thesis.
- There are studies which demonstrate the need for at least a differentiated assessment. In Uganda, the country which thus far has succeeded most in reducing HIV infection rates, there are indications that it was not condom use which played the decisive role, but rather reduction in the number of sexual partners (Stoneburner 2000).
- A large-scale study compared four cities in four African countries (Kenya, Zambia, Cameroon and Benin) with very different HIV preva-

> Theoretically, the use of condoms can prevent HIV transmission by almost 100 per cent. In reality, however, "use errors" and so on reduce effective protection to 85 per cent.

lences. The result was that the spread of HIV was completely independent of the level of condom use (Lagarde et al. 2001).
- A further study in Uganda showed that condom use was relatively low (21 per cent occasionally and 4.4 per cent always) and that consistent condom use definitely lowered the risk of HIV infection. It was remarkable, however, that, with only occasional use, no protective effect against HIV could be found, and the risk of other STIs (chlamydia, gonorrhoea) even increased significantly (Ahmed et al. 2001).
- In sum, condoms offer effective protection against HIV. Correct and consistent use of condoms leads to a decrease in HIV transmission rates.
- However, the significance of condoms in HIV prevention should not be overstated. They are an important component in comprehensive programmes, but taken on their own they can have only a limited impact on the course of the epidemic.
- Cultural and religious reservations about condom use must be taken seriously, since reduction of sexual partners plays at least as great a role. However, the churches should acknowledge their responsibility not to make unscientific assertions and not to stop people from consistently using condoms.
- The availability of male condoms differs from country to country, and also within a given country. According to one study, access to condoms is relatively satisfactory in South Africa, since they can be procured via health facilities (HSCR 2002), but on the whole the general situation is certainly not satisfactory. Approximately 6 billion condoms are distributed every year, but that is only a small fraction of the number of condoms which are actually necessary (UNAIDS 2001a). Thus, one cannot proceed on the assumption that, on the whole, enough condoms are available, and that the low rate of use is due only to non-acceptance.
- Besides the free market, condoms are also available via social marketing (i.e. subsidized) and to a limited degree are also available free of charge. Nevertheless, they are still relatively expensive. Under conditions of poverty, the little money many people have is devoted first of all to day-to-day survival. For many people, the oft-cited claim "I might die of AIDS in 10 years, but I'm starving today" has a very real foundation.

11.6.2 Female condoms

- Women are often more willing than men to use condoms. However, they also frequently have greater difficulties in getting them to be used, since many men refuse.
- In this situation, female condoms have the advantage that they could lead to a greater independence of women in the sexual relationship, since here – in contrast to condoms for men – the women are not (or in any case, are less) dependent on the cooperation of their partner.
- Acceptance of female condoms was not very high in the first years of availability, since they were in part experienced as even more "foreign" than male condoms. However, this appears to be changing. Many projects which work with women discuss the application of these condoms and seek possibilities for receiving information and for promoting their use.

> Correct and consistent use of condoms leads to lower HIV transmission rates. Although the significance of condoms should not be overstated (since reduction in the number of sexual partners plays a role which is at least as great), churches must fulfil their responsibility and not impede people from a consistent use of condoms.

> Compared to the number of condoms which are necessary, the number actually available is quite low.

> Female condoms can lead to an increased self-determination of women in sexual relations, and thus increase protection against HIV infection.

- Female condoms require a high degree of counselling and assistance with respect to proper use. An obstacle preventing a greater dissemination of female condoms is their high price.

11.6.3 Attitude about condoms

- It is often argued that condoms – including for the purposes of family planning – were unknown in traditional society and that they are something artificial and disruptive of the sexual relationship. This argument certainly has its legitimacy. However, it can be used to evade confrontation with HIV. For many men, using condoms puts their masculinity into doubt, and they therefore reject them.
- Reproduction, as an essential function of sexuality, is impeded by the use of condoms. The argument that HIV-infected people would do better not to have children, since the latter would run a high risk of HIV infection and are likely to become orphans, does not correspond to the realities of life for most people, for whom children are an essential component of a fulfilled life. In many traditions, moreover, children are the guarantees that one will live on after death, so that a life without one's own children appears unimaginable. In any case, most people do not know their own HIV status.

> Another obstacle in the use of condoms – besides religious and cultural arguments – is the fact that they interfere with reproduction as an essential function of sexuality.

- For many people, condoms are associated with prostitution and extra-marital and pre-marital sexual relations. Many women and men prefer not to use condoms because, were they to do so, they could be suspected of having extra-marital relationships. This leads to doubts about marital faithfulness and to a loss of trust, a path down which many partners do not want to go. For women, the risk here is even greater, since in their eyes extra-marital sex is generally regarded as undesired and immoral – in contrast to the way the extra-marital relationships of men are generally looked at. Such relations often move women into the proximity of "prostitutes", both in their own eyes and in those of the community.
- Here, prevention messages that condoms should at least be used with extra-marital partners – regardless of the good intentions behind them – certainly have a negative influence on the use of condoms between marital partners. On the other hand, one must question the attitude of some churches, which allow the use of condoms only within marriage, but not in extra-marital relationships, meaning de facto that extra-marital sexual partners have no claim to protection against HIV infection. One proceeds here on the assumption that anything which may not be, simply cannot be.
- Many (married) couples have a discordant HIV status (i.e. one of the partners is HIV-positive and the other HIV-negative). A greater tolerance on the issue of condom use dominates in this case. Many churches approve condoms in the event of discordant HIV status, since they are necessary for protecting the HIV-negative partner against infection. However, since most people do not know their HIV status, they also know nothing of a possible HIV discordance. The general rejection of condoms even for married couples, propagated by several churches, will lead to the HIV-negative partner becoming infected with HIV.

> The general rejection of condoms, as propagated by several churches, thus leaves the HIV-negative partner – in a relationship between partners with discordant HIV status – unprotected against an HIV infection.

– Condom acceptance depends on a series of factors, as presented above. A study conducted in 2002 in South Africa found that condoms are increasingly used: 57 per cent of male and 46 per cent of female 15–24 year olds acknowledged having used condoms during their most recent sexual intercourse. Higher levels of condom use were also associated with higher-risk behaviour: persons with more than one partner in the last year had a greater probability of using condoms than persons with only one sexual partner. Moreover, condom use had risen compared to 1998: earlier, it was still 19.5 per cent for 15–19 year olds and 7.6 per cent for 20–24 year olds. The study attributes increased condom use to promotion of condoms via government campaigns and the relatively widespread availability of condoms in health facilities. But it also found that only 33 per cent of HIV-positive people who knew of their HIV status used condoms (HSRC 2002).

11.7 Male circumcision

> There are indications that male circumcision could reduce the risk of HIV infection. Further studies must be conducted before conclusive recommendations can be given.

– There are indications that male circumcision offers a certain protection against HIV transmission. Thus, one study found that the rates of circumcision in cities with lower HIV prevalence were very much higher than in cities with higher prevalence (Auvert et al. 2001).
– In several regions circumcision is already being advocated and performed as a part of HIV prevention. However, problems can develop during these interventions:
  • Care must be taken to prevent HIV transmission that can occur through the use of unsterilized instruments.
  • Since circumcision can offer only a relative protection against HIV infection, the promotion of this strategy must not foster a false sense of security among affected persons, which in turn could lead to a possibly higher risk of HIV transmission.
– More conclusive results can be expected from further studies currently underway. In the event that indications of the protective function of circumcision are confirmed, a relatively simple and cost-effective method would thus be available as a component of HIV prevention.

11.8 Microbicides

> Nonoxynol-9 has not fulfilled the hopes placed in microbicides. Tests with seaweed and other substances are planned or underway.

– Microbicides are intended to be applied locally in the vagina or rectum and thus to reduce the transmission of sexually transmitted diseases, including HIV. No microbicides are available yet, but there are more than 60 candidates being tested.
– Nonoxynol-9, which for years was regarded as being the most promising, has not lived up to expectations, since a large-scale study among CSWs has shown that it not only does not reduce HIV transmission, but (when used frequently) can even increase it (Van Damme et al. 2002).
– Tests with seaweed and other potential microbicides are planned or already underway.

11.9 PREVENTION AND TREATMENT OF TUBERCULOSIS

- Almost 2 billion people around the world are infected with tuberculosis (TB). However, this does not necessarily mean that they are sick with TB, but rather that they carry the TB bacilli in a dormant state in their bodies. Between 5–10 per cent of these infected people will ultimately really fall ill with TB sometime in their lives: 2 million people die of TB each year.

- The likelihood of falling ill with TB is 30 times higher among people who are infected with both TB and HIV. In 1999 there were almost 2 million new TB cases in Africa, and the majority of them were HIV-positive. Tuberculosis is the primary opportunistic infection in Africa, and the most frequent cause of death among HIV-infected persons. In some countries up to 60 per cent of all TB patients are HIV-positive. If no appropriate measures are forthcoming, TB cases will probably double in Africa within the next decade due to the HIV epidemic and the lack of financing for more effective strategies to fight tuberculosis (UNAIDS 2001e).

- TB and HIV should be combated together in control programmes, since reduction of HIV transmission would also have an impact on the TB epidemic.

- TB is much more infectious than HIV. It can also be transmitted through household contact, since the tubercle bacilli can be spread by coughing. This creates a high risk that tuberculosis is transmitted to HIV-negative people in the vicinity of TB patients.

- In contrast to HIV, TB is curable. WHO recommends treating TB according to the DOTS scheme (directly observed treatment – short course). This means a minimum 6-month course with a combination of drugs which are taken under the supervision of a health worker or a member of the community or family. The DOTS scheme also entails that the treatment with TB drugs be guaranteed, which often represents a special problem in countries with inadequate healthcare infrastructures, and that there be a political commitment to implementation (WHO 2000).

- Monitoring of therapy is included as an important component, in order to avoid patients stopping treatment after initial improvement of symptoms, which is generally experienced. Since HIV-infected people develop drug-resistant forms of TB especially frequently, careful observation of the therapy and adequate treatment with drugs are imperative.

- Studies have determined that TB prophylaxis with Isoniazid for people who are infected with HIV is effective. WHO and UNAIDS have concluded that such a prophylaxis forms part of a package of treatment options which should be available to HIV-infected persons, although it is not an alternative to treating TB according to the DOTS scheme (WHO/UNAIDS 1998).

> In Africa TB is the most frequent opportunistic infection. HIV-infected people run a much higher risk of getting TB, which is causing TB infection to spread rapidly in countries with high HIV prevalence.

11.10 Treatment of sexually transmitted infections (STIs)

> STIs are widespread in poor countries, above all due to the lack of healthcare. Since they substantially increase the risk of HIV transmission, treatment of STIs is of great importance in HIV prevention.

- In general, poorer countries have a higher rate of sexually transmitted infections than do rich industrialized countries. This is because their lack of healthcare facilities means diseases are inadequately diagnosed and treated. STIs such as syphilis, gonorrhoea, etc., are co-factors in HIV transmission. This means that the presence of one of these diseases, above all when they are coupled with ulcerative skin changes, increases the risk of HIV transmission through sexual contact.

- Various studies are therefore investigating how, under conditions of limited resources, an effective and efficient treatment of STIs is possible. A study in Tanzania showed a 38 per cent reduction in HIV incidence when STIs were treated on the basis of symptoms (syndromic management) and health centres were adequately equipped (Grosskurth et al. 1995). Another study in Uganda, however, found no decline in HIV incidence under mass treatment of STIs (Wawer et al. 1999). There are several explanatory models for these divergent results, such as different sexual behaviour and different HIV prevalences at baseline (Grosskurth et al. 2000). Above all, infections with herpes simplex virus-2 probably play a major role in HIV transmission, as is being increasingly recognized (Laga et al. 2001). There is however no causal treatment for these viral infections.

- In conclusion, the treatment of STIs plays an important role in HIV prevention.

11.11 Blood transfusions

> Since the risk of HIV transmission in the event of transfusing HIV-infected blood is >90%, adequate and safe blood transfusion practices in health facilities are vitally important.

- The risk that HIV is transmitted during a transfusion with infected blood is >90%, since with this type of transmission the virus arrives in massive quantities directly in the bloodstream.

- An unknown number of people are infected with HIV via infected blood. Affected above all are children and pregnant women, who run a higher risk of anaemias (lack of blood due to malaria and other diseases) which require a blood transfusion.

- Some developing countries have properly functioning blood bank systems in hospitals, which screen all blood transfusion products for HIV. In several countries, administering such a test is still not the rule before a transfusion, or it is not adequately performed. A study in Kenya revealed that in 1994 the HIV prevalence among blood donors was 6.4 per cent. HIV was transmitted in approximately 2 per cent of the transfusions performed, primarily due to poor laboratory practices. After learning of these results, the Kenyan Health Ministry undertook a series of interventions to improve the situation (Moore et al. 2001).

- In many places, patients are now only transfused when, without a transfusion, they would die from lack of blood. This practice offers an additional protection against HIV infection, since even with screening of transfusion products there still exists a low risk that – due to the window period – the blood to be transfused is infected with HIV.

- Screening of blood and blood products in health facilities therefore plays a major role in HIV prevention.

11.12 Vaccine research

- For years it has been rightly emphasized that an effective vaccine against HIV would provide the best hope for stopping its worldwide spread. Thus, the question is constantly posed: will there be an AIDS vaccine and, if so, when?

- Research is difficult for bio-chemical reasons: the structure of the virus is constantly changing, and HIV attacks the very cells that are responsible for the immune defence in the human body.

- There are also political reasons: incentives for the industry to invest money in this research field have been low. Companies know that the vaccine is most needed precisely where people have the least money to pay for it.

- Organizations such as the World Bank and the EU are working out how public funds can be used to increase incentives for vaccine research. The possibilities being discussed include an international fund from which the eventual product can be made available at a low price to poorer countries. Private organizations (e.g. International AIDS Vaccine Initiative and the Bill Gates Foundation) are making more funds available and are engaging in advocacy work.

- Intensive work is necessary right now so that a potential vaccine can then be made available as quickly as possible to the people who need it most urgently (Esparza 2001).

- A number of vaccine candidates are being tested in phase 1, 2 and 3 trials. Two phase 3 trials (that is, field tests with thousands of volunteers) were undertaken in the US and Thailand. The results of the Thai trial were published in November 2003 and showed no protective effect of the vaccine given when compared to the group that had received placebos (McCarthy 2003).

- These trials relate to the virus subtypes B and E, which appear predominantly in Europe, North America and Southeast Asia. Results for the subtypes which predominate in Africa are expected at a later time.

- Up till now, attempts have been made to find a vaccine which prevents cells from being infected with the virus, but more recent efforts seek to reduce transmission immunotherapeutically, by strengthening immune defence.

- In the scientific sense, vaccine research has made considerable progress over the last decade, and various strategies are being pursued. However, it is probable that no vaccine will be 100 per cent effective. Although it is likely to exert an essential influence on the course of the epidemic, other prevention methods will still be necessary.

- Even in a best-case scenario, it will still be several years before a vaccine can be marketed. This process could be accelerated through stronger support for the promising approaches via public funding.

> Vaccine research is made more difficult (on the biological level) since the structure of the virus is constantly changing, and (on the political level) because the incentives for the industry to invest in this area of research are low.

> It is likely that no vaccine will ever be 100 per cent effective, and so other prevention methods will still be required. Moreover, even under the most favourable assumptions, the introduction is still years away.

12. Mother-to-child HIV transmission (MTCT)

12.1 Risk reduction

In Africa, the risk of vertical transmission of HIV is 25–45 per cent.

- The overall risk that, without interventions, there will be vertical transmission from mother to child amounts to 25–45 per cent (UNICEF/WHO/UNAIDS 1998a). This can take place at different points in time. Around one-half of transmissions occur during pregnancy and birth, the other half during the breastfeeding period (Newell 1998).

- MTCT is also called parent-to-child transmission (PTCT) to avoid blaming mothers for infecting their children, since the great majority of cases also involve a male who has in the first place infected the woman.

- There are various options for decreasing the risk of vertical HIV transmission. First, there is primary prevention among women (i.e. the prevention of an HIV infection among women in the reproductive phase). A second option is family planning among already HIV-infected women (i.e. women who know their HIV status should receive access to counselling and contraception).

- In principle, HIV-positive women in industrialized countries who require antiretroviral therapy continue to receive it during pregnancy. This lowers the risk of transmission to the child. If they themselves are not receiving antiretroviral therapy, during the birth they receive either AZT or Nevirapine (likewise two antiretroviral drugs) in a dosage which only has an effect on the transmission to the child.

The drug Nevirapine can reduce the risk of vertical transmission by 50%.

- A study with Nevirapine in Uganda showed that, by giving this medication, the overall risk of HIV infection after 14–16 weeks of life amounted to only 13 per cent for the children, which corresponds to a reduction of 50 per cent in comparison to the group that was not treated. In the study, the mother received only one tablet of Nevirapine (200mg) during delivery and the child received one dose (2mg/kg) after the birth. The transmission rate reduced by half and was achieved despite the fact that the children were breastfed until the 12th week of life (Guay et al. 1999). A long-term follow-up of the study showed that the survival benefit persisted up to 18 months of age. Infants who had received Nevirapine had significantly lower risk of HIV infection than those who received AZT (15.7 per cent vs. 25.8 per cent) (Brooks Jackson et al. 2003).

- Since July 2001 the drug Nevirapine has been donated by the manufacturer Boehringer/Ingelheim free of charge to developing countries in order to reduce mother-to-child transmission. However, this donation does not relate to the use of Nevirapine in antiretroviral therapy, but only for the indication of reduction of mother-to-child transmission.

- However, giving Nevirapine to HIV-positive pregnant women requires significant additional resources for HIV tests and counselling of the pregnant women, which affected countries cannot easily afford. In Africa, only 1 per cent of all pregnant women receive voluntary counselling and testing.

- There are increasing demands that ARV therapy also be made available for mothers (and the rest of the family) whenever necessary. This is known as MTCT+ (mother-to-child transmission plus). This is desirable for several reasons:

- It is being considered for ethical reasons. When giving Nevirapine, the mother receives the drugs only to prevent HIV transmission to the child, but thereafter gets no further ARV therapy for herself (i.e. the course of her disease is not altered in any positive way) and she is likely to die from AIDS in the future.
- Treating mothers with life-prolonging ARV therapy will also prevent children from becoming orphans.
- There are growing concerns about resistances to Nevirapine that may occur even after a single dose application, as in the reduction of mother-to-child transmission. This would then render Nevirapine and similar drugs useless in the treatment of women and children (if they were to receive ARV therapy later). Since Nevirapine is very often given as a first-line drug, this has potentially severe implications for ARV therapy on a larger scale. Calls are being made for other ARV drugs to be added to Nevirapine to avoid resistances or, better still, that mothers who need ARV therapy receive it. Further research and policy changes are urgently required (Palmore Beckham 2003).

> There are increasing demands that ARV therapy also be made available for mothers themselves (and the rest of the family) whenever necessary. The practice of giving drugs only to reduce the transmission to the child will not alter the course of the mother's HIV disease positively.

12.2 PROBLEMS FOR AFFECTED WOMEN

- For women to learn during pregnancy of their HIV infection (and possibly to be exposed to discrimination and violence) means an additional burden at a crucial time. Counselling and drugs to reduce transmission to the child are therefore sometimes not utilized, even when they are available.
- Traditionally, all women in Africa and other regions have breastfed, and this practice is still the norm today, at least in rural areas. A stigma is attached to other forms of feeding, and this frequently exposes women to the suspicion that they are HIV-positive. Data from Uganda show that 60–80 per cent of HIV-positive women decided to breastfeed after they had been counselled on the risk of transmitting HIV, mainly due to fear of the social stigma (Maman et al. 2001).
- After the experience of seeing their child suffer and die, many women decide against having another child anyway.
- Mothers should not be blamed for either transmitting HIV to their child through breastfeeding or of having caused the child's death through malnutrition by not breastfeeding.
- The influence of families and communities on the decisions of women must also be taken into account here, and general education about HIV within communities is required. The role of men and fathers must be reconsidered in this connection. In many settings, when women come to a clinic for delivery, the father of the child cannot be found and identified immediately. Nevertheless, the influence of these fathers is perceptible, and is expressed in women's lack of decision-making power.

> Pregnant women who are HIV-positive must be protected against further stigmatization and attribution of guilt.

12.3 CURRENT RECOMMENDATIONS

- An important aspect of breastfeeding risk is the manner of breastfeeding: is the child nourished exclusively with breast milk, or is supplementary nourishment also given? A prospective study from South Africa was able to identify increased HIV transmission only among children who were not exclusively breastfed (overall risk after 3 months: 24 per cent). By contrast, exclusively breastfed children had a risk comparable to children who were immediately weaned after birth (14.6 per cent versus 18.8 per cent, a statistically insignificant difference) (Coutsoudis et al. 1999). It is suspected that giving formula feeding together with breast milk cumulates the negative consequences: an exposure to the virus with simultaneously reduced immune defence (through contaminated water etc. in the supplementary diet).

- Modification of breastfeeding behaviour can reduce transmission during the breastfeeding period. There are several alternatives:
  - Not breastfeeding is generally recommended to HIV-positive women in settings with affordable and practicable alternatives to mother's milk (e.g. infant formula feeding).
  - Early weaning, at the latest after the sixth month of life.
  - Intensive breastfeeding counselling which highlights the importance of exclusive breastfeeding.

- To implement these recommendations, various alternatives for early-childhood nutrition have been proposed (UNICEF/WHO/UNAIDS 1998b). These include commercially produced infant formula, self-production with locally available products (e.g. from fresh animal milk or milk powder, breast milk from which the HI virus has been eliminated by heat treatment – 30 minutes at 62.5°C), milk banks and wet-nursing.

- UNICEF, WHO and UNAIDS, which essentially co-define the guidelines for health measures in developing countries, issued the following guidelines in 1998 (UNICEF/WHO/UNAIDS 1998b):
  - All women should have the right and the possibility of learning their HIV status.
  - All women who are infected with HIV should be informed about the options to reduce the risk of vertical transmission.
  - For all women who are not HIV-infected or who do not know their status there applies a general recommendation to breastfeed.
  - All HIV-infected women should receive individual counselling, in which all possible alternatives to breastfeeding are discussed.
  - The decision of the woman must then be supported in any case.

- All efforts must be undertaken in order to retain, even among HIV-infected mothers, the life-promoting method of breastfeeding and to keep the potential dangers as low as possible. It is feared that, if non-breastfeeding is propagated too widely, this practice will also catch on among HIV-negative mothers. This would probably result in increased child mortality. A role in these discussions is also played by the producers of infant formula food, who have an interest in the distribution and sale of their products.

> All women should have the right and the possibility to learn about their HIV status and should be informed about the options for reducing the risk of HIV transmission to the baby.

- These recommendations must be understood as general guidelines which, under the given economic and cultural conditions in many countries, cannot be implemented simply like that. In order to take this problem into account and to consider the most recent scientific knowledge, an expert group headed by the WHO further refined the guidelines of 1998 (WHO Technical Consultation 2001):
  - It is to be recommended that HIV-infected mothers avoid breastfeeding, when adequate, affordable, sustainable and safe alternatives are available.
  - Otherwise, exclusive breastfeeding for the first months of life is recommended.
  - The best point in time for shifting from exclusive breastfeeding to weaning cannot be generally established, and depends on the local context.
  - Studies should be performed to assess the best nutritional options for infants after the breastfeeding period within the local context.
  - An adequate number of skilled workers should be trained who can provide good breastfeeding and nutritional counselling for HIV-infected women.

> When adequate, affordable, sustainable and safe alternatives are available, one should recommend to HIV-positive mothers to avoid breastfeeding. Otherwise, exclusive breastfeeding for the first months of life, with relatively early weaning, is recommended.

13. Care

13.1 CONTINUUM OF CARE

> People affected by HIV need comprehensive care. The various areas which provide care and treatment must form a continuum of care.

- People living with HIV/AIDS need medical, nursing, spiritual, psychological, social and material care. This must be embedded in a continuum of care in which the various formal and informal services which provide care (hospitals, home care, social services, support groups) are linked in a network. Voluntary counselling and testing frequently serves as an entry into this system (Osborne 1996).

- Individual components must not be seen in isolation, or as in competition with one another. Instead, they should complement one another, as each has its specific legitimacy and role in HIV/AIDS treatment.

- Medical care and treatment of HIV/AIDS in poor countries includes in principle the same care as in rich countries, since the illness (in medical respects) is fundamentally identical. A decisive difference lies in the inadequate access of most people in poor countries to drugs and care in general, so that, for individuals, getting sick is a much more serious matter.

- Dying of HIV/AIDS (or of the chronic illnesses associated with AIDS) is often a process which goes on for years, during which time people become sick repeatedly, with periods of improvement in between. As the disease advances, the episodes of illness increase in frequency and severity, conditioned by the progressive collapse of the immune system. Patients often have several symptoms or illnesses simultaneously, such as chronic coughing and difficulty in breathing, diarrhoea, an itching and painful skin rash and vomiting. Many patients have chronic pain (e.g. during or after a herpes zoster illness), which can severely interfere with life. The patient's forces gradually decline and periods of confinement in bed increase. Without access to adequate therapy, those affected also realize that death is unavoidable, and they are further burdened by concerns for the fate of the surviving family.

13.2 INTERDEPENDENCE OF PREVENTION AND CARE

> Fighting AIDS must include the three interdependent areas of prevention, care and mitigation of impact.

- An effective response to the challenge of HIV/AIDS must include:
  - Reduction of the number of new infections (prevention).
  - Provision of treatment and care.
  - Mitigation of the social, political and economic impact of the epidemic.

- These three areas are interdependent: care and prevention must be considered as a whole. They belong together in the reality of the people who are affected. Scarcity of resources and the expertise which is necessary for many programmes can make it necessary for HIV/AIDS interventions to place the focus on a single component. When developing and implementing a programme, however, the interdependence of the various areas must be taken into account.

- The social consequences of the HIV epidemic increase vulnerability to HIV infection and make HIV prevention more difficult (Piot and Coll-Seck 2001).
- Caring for HIV-infected persons and those affected by HIV has positive effects on prevention. People are more willing to undergo an HIV test if they know that, in the event of HIV infection, they will receive adequate treatment.
- HIV interventions which aim exclusively at prevention lack credibility and are unacceptable for people. As long as knowledge about one's own HIV infection leads to a multitude of disadvantages such as stigma and lack of treatment, then at least some of the care continuum must be associated with each prevention programme.
- For the individual person, prevention of HIV illness is always preferable to treatment. However, once infection or illness has occurred, treatment and care must also be provided for ethical and moral reasons.
- Jesus Christ commanded us to love our neighbours and to serve them, which makes a commitment on the part of the churches necessary in this respect.
- In order to reduce vulnerability to HIV infection, one must change the social factors which create such vulnerability: thus, promotion of gender equity, reduction of poverty, provision of basic school education for everyone, etc., are vital.

13.3 Home-based care

- In many countries home-based care initiatives have emerged, often within the framework of churches. Home-based care strives for comprehensive care of those who are affected by HIV: assistance in caring for family members, help with the housework, transport of patients to and from hospital, provision of nursing aids (soap, sheets and so on), aid with funerals, care for orphans and other survivors, material assistance (e.g. with food), distribution of medications. Frequently, however, one seeks the collaboration of trained medical personnel, either as volunteers or operating from health facilities. Some home care programmes have also begun with the treatment and supervision of tuberculosis therapy.
- A wide range of different initiatives and programmes are included under the concept of home care. Given the full extent of the epidemic, however, their scope and coverage is by no means adequate. Home care is essentially borne by NGOs and community groups, in particular the churches, and on the whole government participation in these programmes is rather low (Nsutebu et al. 2001).

  > Widely differing initiatives are included under the denominator of home care. In general, however, it is borne mainly by NGOs, and to a great extent by the churches.

- Caring for and visiting the sick are an important part of most traditional societies. Caring for the sick was and still is largely performed by female family members. Women also form the majority in home care groups.
- This increases the workload and the psychological stress on women. On the other hand, there is a possibility for the empowerment of individual women and groups. In the home care initiatives, new skills (e.g. counselling and nursing) are learned and applied, which can increase the

  > The vast majority of volunteers in home care are women. This can lead to greater self-confidence on the part of women, but it also raises the danger that women will be overworked.

autonomy of participants. For reasons of workload and the equal rights and duties of men and women, however, many projects are seeking a higher participation of men in home care work.

- Great significance is attributed to home care because the health systems in many poor countries are chronically understaffed and they cannot deal with the additional burden caused by the HIV epidemic. Here, community-based home care, in contrast to hospital-based home care, offered itself, so to speak, as the cheaper alternative. Follow-up was initially conducted in the homes of the patients by hospital-based care services (hospital-based home care). Then these tasks were frequently organized and performed by communities themselves (community-based home care). Hospital-based care is more expensive than community-based care. As in other areas, here, too, communities should be involved as much as possible.

- If home care is to be more than merely visiting the patients, it needs resources: for training of volunteers, basic medications and the social support of the (mostly very poor) patients and their families (means of transport, fees for hospital treatment and drugs). The necessary resources are often underestimated.

- Each programme should have a sufficient number of trained volunteers. Here, a few weeks of training in basic counselling, nursing, etc. can often be enough for a start. Refresher training is necessary during the course of the work. In planning, at the start or even during the course of a home care programme, links should be established with other comparable programmes in order to learn from one another through information exchange and visits.

- Many initiatives also have a component for the care of orphans. Subsidies in the form of money or food are given to families and school fees are paid so that orphans can continue to attend school (or go to one for the first time).

- The issue of payment or financial incentives for volunteers is often discussed. It is argued that payment would remove the character of neighbourhood assistance or Christian love of the neighbour. Many of those who are active as volunteers in home care, however, contribute significantly to family income. This particularly concerns women volunteers, many of whom work in the informal sector. Women, moreover, have work in the household which demands a significant amount of time. Thus, significant social costs are generated for those participating in home care. At the very least one should provide incentives such as clothing and coverage of costs in the event of illness, etc. for volunteers.

Home care lightens the burden on hospitals and helps to destigmatize HIV/AIDS. In order to do their job adequately, home care programmes must have sufficient resources.

- Compared to hospital care of chronic patients, home care offers several advantages:

  - It contributes to relieving the pressure on overburdened, under-equipped and understaffed hospitals.
  - Many patients prefer care at home to care in hospital.
  - Communities are integrated into the care of the chronically sick. This helps destigmatize AIDS, breaks down denial, and thus aids prevention of HIV/AIDS.

- Churches have already made a great contribution to promoting projects in these areas. Churches and other organizations should not implement home care programmes for communities; rather, communities should themselves carry out the programmes. This is more effective, more efficient, and moreover contributes to the empowerment of communities.
- However, the establishment of home care programmes must not lead to a situation where necessary investments in health facilities are omitted and all of the nursing burdens are imposed on communities, especially on women. Home care is not a cheap form of care for those affected by HIV. The programmes must therefore have enough resources available to perform their tasks adequately.

13.4 Hospitals and health centres

- Through hospitals and health centres, churches in developing countries provide a large share of healthcare. With the HIV epidemic, these tasks have become even more vital, since hospitals often are no longer able to cope with the increasing numbers of patients and guarantee good-quality care for the sick.
- On the basis of their infrastructure, resources and access to broad parts of the population, church health facilities are in a position to take over responsibility for essential tasks in the fight against HIV:
  - Organization of and/or involvement in home care implemented by communities.
  - HIV education (e.g. for pregnant women, mothers, young people).
  - Treatment of sexually transmitted infections (as prevention of HIV transmission).
  - Voluntary HIV counselling and testing.
  - Treatment of HIV-associated diseases and opportunistic infections.
  - Provision of life-prolonging antiretroviral therapy.
- Church health facilities bear a special responsibility since, on the basis of their option for the poor, they offer what for many people – given the impoverishment caused by AIDS – is their sole access to health services.

> In developing countries, churches provide a large proportion of healthcare. They bear a special responsibility, since – given the impoverishment caused by AIDS – for many people they constitute the sole source of healthcare.

13.5 Hospices

- In several countries, hospices have developed which care for the chronically ill and dying. Some hospices admit patients or offer a more humane way to die; others are day centres for HIV-positive people, from which health personnel operate in home care.
- In many situations there is an understandable wish to be able to offer care in a hospice, so that death can take place in respectful and suitable surroundings.
- Hospices are also places where the chronically ill, who at home may be close to death due to lack of care, can recover and survive.
- However, hospices which offer institutionalized care are relatively expensive. In addition, they remove the chronically sick from their environ-

> To avoid the establishment of expensive hospices (on an in-patient basis), communities and families should be supported in their resources, so that the sick and dying can be cared for at home.

ment. Therefore, for the chronically ill and the dying, care at home is preferable. For this, families and communities must be strengthened in their capacities, so that they can take over responsibility for care. In situations where no family is present any longer, all possibilities of searching for a family, a foster family or reintegration of the patient into the family must be exhausted.

13.6 TRADITIONAL MEDICINE

– In many countries, traditional medicine remains very important. Most people consult both "Western" health facilities and traditional healers. Some countries have achieved successes in integrating traditional healers into HIV programmes: the healers speak to their patients about AIDS, work together with health institutions and become aware of the risk of HIV transmission when using instruments which come into contact with the blood of patients.

– For example, the Bamalete Lutheran Hospital in Botswana has a programme in which traditional healers work closely with hospital doctors in fighting AIDS, and a system of mutual referrals has been established.

– There are no reliable data on what risk exists due to the use of treatment instruments in traditional medicine, such as in connection with tattooing, and of the risk of HIV infection through these interventions. Nor are there enough data on successful approaches to treating opportunistic infections with traditional medicine, which undoubtedly exist.

– Traditional healers have great potential in the fight against AIDS, which in many places has not yet been fully considered.

> Traditional healers have a major responsibility and also great potential in the fight against AIDS, something which in many places has not yet been sufficiently recognized.

14. Antiretroviral therapy

14.1 ANTIRETROVIRAL DRUGS (ARV)

- In industrialized countries, combination therapy with antiretroviral drugs has been used to treat HIV infections since 1996. ARV drugs act specifically against the HI virus. They are subdivided into several classes. Since the introduction of combination ARV therapy, death rates from AIDS have fallen by as much as 70 per cent in the rich countries.

- NRTI (nucleoside reverse transcriptase inhibitors), NNRTI (non-nucleoside reverse transcriptase inhibitors) and PI (protease inhibitors) are used. They largely suppress virus replication, slow down the disease course, and lower illness frequency and death rates if they are taken in combinations of at least three drugs (in part from different classes). This so-called HAART (Highly Active Antiretroviral Therapy) applies for all countries, and deviation from this standard is not allowed for medical reasons.

- There is a need for the development of new drugs and drug classes, since resistances are developing against the existing ones. The first representative of a new ARV class, the fusion inhibitors, was approved in the US in 2003.

- ARV are usually not taken from the start of the infection, but rather only when the infection has reached a certain stage. Since HIV/AIDS is fatal without treatment in virtually all cases, sooner or later all HIV infected persons must receive these drugs if death is to be prevented.

- WHO has issued guidelines which also apply for use in resource-poor countries. Thus, ARV should in any case be given in the AIDS stage, and/or when the CD4 cell count has fallen below 200/µl. In the resource-rich countries, therapy monitoring also includes laboratory determination of the CD4 cells and determination of viral load, which is a measure of the number of virus in the blood. These measurements should as far as possible be performed even under more limited resource conditions; however, the lack of resources for their implementation should not hinder the introduction of ARV therapy (WHO 2002a).

> In the first years after introduction of the effective combination therapy in 1996, access to these drugs was not regarded as a realistic option for poor countries. This view has been rethought, however: ARV programmes are effective and can be implemented even with limited resources, drug prices have fallen, and moral–ethical concerns are making the gap in AIDS treatment worldwide increasingly unacceptable.

14.2 ACCESS TO ARV

<1% of PLWHA in Africa have access to ARV therapy.

– Of the 800,000 people globally who take ARV drugs, around 500,000 live in industrialized countries. The following table gives the actual and estimated need for ARV therapy in developing countries (ITAC 2002):

Region	No of people on ARV therapy	Estimated need	Coverage
Sub-Saharan Africa	50,000	4,100,000	1%
Asia	43,000	1,000,000	4%
Northern Africa & Middle East	3,000	7,000	29%
Eastern Europe & Central Asia	7,000	80,000	9%
Latin America & Caribbean	196,000	370,000	53%
Total	**300,000**	**5,500,000**	**5%**

Of the 800,000 people globally who take ARV drugs, around 500,000 live in the industrialized countries.

– Initially, access to ARV drugs for poor countries was often not regarded as a realistic option. The high prices of the drugs, patent protection for brand-name drugs, inadequate infrastructure and lack of training of healthcare workers in the affected poor countries were seen as blocking access to ARV.

– However, in recent years the demand to increase access to ARV for PLWHA in the developing countries has been raised ever more loudly by AIDS activists, scientists and civil society. A first essential contribution came from a group of scientists at Harvard University, who in 2001 presented an implementation and financing plan for the broad introduction of medical treatment of AIDS in Africa (Individual Members of the Faculty of Harvard University 2001).

– Since then, a change in thinking has taken place which is conditioned by the increased awareness for the ethical–moral implications of inequality in AIDS treatment between poor and rich countries, as well as by the fact that implementation of corresponding programmes is a realistic option: the prices for ARV drugs have fallen substantially, and a number of pilot projects have shown that ARV treatment programmes are effective and feasible under conditions of limited resources.

– In the successfully implemented programmes (e.g. by a Harvard University group in Haiti and government programmes in Senegal and Uganda), the clinical and biological results of ARV are comparable to those in corresponding populations in industrialized countries (Farmer et al. 2001; Laurent et al. 2002; Weidle et al. 2002).

– The same result was also found by Médecins sans Frontières (Doctors Without Borders), which has been implementing an ARV project in a poor suburb of Cape Town, in collaboration with the Treatment Action Campaign. The results show that for 90 per cent of the patients the viral load fell below the detection limit, that adherence (as a measure for regularly taking the tablets) is very good, and that clinical parameters, such as increase in weight and reduction of the opportunistic diseases and side effects of the drugs, correspond to those in the Western countries (Kasper et al. 2002).

– The issue of access to ARV for people in developing countries is not a medical, but rather a political question: the medical treatment of HIV infection follows the same principles throughout the world.

– Access to comprehensive care and treatment is not an optional luxury in the global response to HIV/AIDS, but rather a necessity in all settings, both rich and poor, and must embrace the full continuum, including home care, palliative care, treatment of opportunistic infections and antiretroviral therapy.

– There are some studies which indicate a rise in new infections due to increased risk behaviour (reduction of safer sex) after introduction of ARV treatment. However, these results were found in specific populations of homosexual men in the industrialized countries, not all studies show these results, and it is not clear whether something similar is also being observed in a heterosexual population. Finally, a life-preserving therapy cannot be withheld from entire populations on the grounds of possibly heightened risk behaviour.

– There have been substantial developments in individual countries and on the global level resulting in increased access to ARV drugs:

  - In January 2002, Botswana became the first African country to implement a programme which provides ARV for all HIV-infected persons (Africa Comprehensive HIV/AIDS Partnership 2002). It is planned to expand the programme in the coming years to all hospitals and to integrate all of the estimated 110,000 HIV-infected persons who require ARV into the programme.

  > In 2002, Botswana became the first African country to begin implementing a programme whose objective is to give universal access to ARV treatment.

  - In August 2003, the South African government declared a roll out of a nationwide programme to increase access to ARV through public health facilities (DOH 2003). The activist movement Treatment Action Campaign had in recent years exerted corresponding pressure on the government, since it had been reluctant to embark on such a programme.

  > In 2003 the South African government declared a roll out of a nationwide programme to increase access to ARV through public health facilities.

  - In Southern Africa, a number of large multinational corporations have started to make ARV treatment available for their workers, sometimes also for their families.

  - In Kenya, churches, field-based organizations (FBOs) and others have trained healthcare workers in ARV therapy management, and in mission and government hospitals thousands of patients are receiving ARV treatment. The government plans a programme for the reduction of mother-to-child transmission and also to increase access to ARV therapy.

  - Money from the the Global Fund to Fight AIDS, Tuberculosis and Malaria is beginning to reach affected countries. For example, Zambia will use funds to finance the introduction of ARV for (initially) 10,000 people. A great proportion of the funds will be disbursed to church-related health facilities.

– Brazil, Argentina, Costa Rica, Cuba and Uruguay have government programmes which should guarantee free universal access to ARV treatment. However, there are major differences in the prices of the drugs in the individual countries, and thus actual access to the drugs also varies.

> Brazil has successfully organized access to ARV treatment for all people living with HIV/AIDS.

- Brazil is seen as an example where, in a middle-income country, universal access to ARV has generated significant savings in the healthcare sector and the number of new infections has remained substantially below the expected figure. These results make the intervention a cost-effective one for Brazil. Brazil has few patents on ARV drugs, and has therefore until now been able to cheaply produce generic drugs itself (UNAIDS 2002).

> WHO's "3 by 5" initiative has the objective of providing access to ARV treatment for 3 million people by the end of 2005.

- WHO declared HIV/AIDS a global health emergency and started its "3 by 5" initiative which plans to give 3 million people access to ARV by the year 2005. To achieve this goal, it will work closely with the Global Fund (www.who.int/).

- The successful implementation of ARV programmes requires a standardized therapy which simplifies the treatment without compromising the therapeutic "gold standards" which apply in the rich countries. A contribution to this effort is made by two WHO documents, which provide recommendations for the proper use of drugs under limited resource conditions and which undertake a quality review of the corresponding brand and generic drugs (WHO 2002a, 2002b). These recommendations are regularly updated.

> In 2002 WHO added antiretroviral drugs to its List of Essential Drugs.

- In April 2002, moreover, WHO decided to add ARV drugs to its List of Essential Drugs. This list, which is recognized as a recommendation throughout the world, had until then included only AZT and Nevirapine for reducing mother-to-child transmission of HIV. WHO is setting new standards by expanding the spectrum of drugs and enlarging the indication for general ARV therapy (WHO 2002c).

- Ecumenical Pharmaceutical Network: see p. 100.

14.3 Drug prices

> Responding to international pressure, multinational pharmaceutical companies have significantly reduced their prices for ARV drugs for Africa.

- At world market prices, ARV drugs cost US$10,000–15,000 per patient per year. Due above all to international pressure and competition from generic drugs, multinational pharmaceutical companies have reduced the prices for ARV for African countries by up to 90 per cent – in some instances, even more.

- The strategy followed thus far of price negotiations by individual countries with multinational pharmaceutical companies has not produced satisfactory results. As is becoming clear in Latin America for example, countries with greater negotiating power can attain substantially more favourable prices than countries with a weaker starting position. Therefore, regional or global arrangements have been proposed, possibly with UN participation, in order to achieve substantial price reductions.

- Producers of generic drugs (e.g. from India) offer corresponding drugs at even more favourable prices, for US$200–350 per patient per year. At the end of 2003, the Clinton Foundation negotiated prices for some developing countries with generic producers for US$130 per patient per

year. But even at these reduced prices the drugs are still not affordable for the overwhelming majority of the people affected.
- Another option for substantial price reductions is differential pricing, where pharmaceutical firms set more favourable prices for the poor and higher prices for the rich countries.
- Médecins sans Frontières publishes a regularly revised list which seeks to disentangle the confusion of prices for ARV drugs, which should help organizations to procure them favourably (MSF 2003).

14.4 PATENTS

- Greater availability of ARV generic drugs is barred by the patent rules of the TRIPS Agreement (Trade Related Aspects of Intellectual Property Rights) of the World Trade Organization (WTO). This grants patent protection for drugs for 20 years (WTO 1994). Thus, it is argued, prices are being kept artificially high, since competition from cheaper generic drugs is being blocked. It is true that not all ARV drugs are patented in Africa, but the drugs which are essential under the conditions of limited resources are affected to a higher than average degree (Attaran and Gillespie-White 2001; Goemare et al. 2002).

> International agreements grant patent protection on drugs for 20 years, thus blocking competition from cheaper generic drugs. The agreements, however, contain rules according to which governments, through compulsory licences, can commission a local firm to produce the corresponding drugs more cheaply.

- The TRIPS Agreement includes safeguards under which, for example, a government can declare a public health emergency and by issuing compulsory licences can authorize local firms to produce the corresponding drugs as generic drugs.
- In one widely noted case, 40 multinational pharmaceutical companies undertook legal steps to compel the South African government to rescind a law which allowed production of generic drugs in South Africa under the special provisions of the TRIPS Agreement. As a result of international protests, the complaint was finally withdrawn in April 2001.
- In a high-profile declaration at its Ministerial Conference in Doha in November 2001, WTO declared that the TRIPS Agreement can and must be interpreted in such a way that it may not impede access to health care, and that countries themselves can define how and under what conditions they wish to apply the safeguards of the Agreement (WTO 2001). This declaration was generally seen as an arrangement favouring the access of poor countries to the corresponding drugs.
- Compulsory licences have not yet found wider application. Political influence exerted by the governments of rich countries and by multinational pharmaceutical companies on developing countries is believed to be responsible for this. There are some countries where by the end of 2003 some progress had been made on this issue (e.g. South Africa and Kenya).
- A further unresolved problem has been access to ARV in the countries which do not have the capacity for producing generic drugs, since compulsory licences generally entitle one only to produce generic drugs for consumption in one's own country. WTO's Doha Declaration called for a solution to this problem by the end of 2002. Under pressure (above all from the US), it was proposed to interpret the Doha Declaration more restrictively, so that it only applies to certain drugs.

> There is resistance to application of the TRIPS safeguards. For example, 40 pharmaceutical companies sued the South African government to block application of these rules. Due to the international protest this provoked, however, it was ultimately decided to withdraw the complaint. Yet the rich countries apply the safeguards in their own interest.

- At the latest by 2005, countries such as India which possess generic drugs production capacity must comply fully with TRIPS. After that date they will no longer be available as generic drugs producers.
- At a WTO meeting prior to the ministerial meeting in Cancun in August 2003, it was resolved that countries could produce generic drugs for export under certain conditions (not for profit, to be specified which country they go to and which quantity, etc.) (WTO 2003). Médecins sans Frontières (2003) and others argue that this is likely to create huge bureaucratic hurdles for the countries that wish to apply the regulations, but that this solution is at least some step forward towards greater access to drugs for poor countries that do not have the capacity to manufacture drugs themselves.
- Industrialized countries are themselves using TRIPS safeguards in their own interests. In September 2001 the US and Canadian governments successfully threatened to apply compulsory licences to meet the anthrax menace. To the announcement that there would be compulsory licences if the medication for treating anthrax was not available in sufficient quantities and at appropriate prices, the producer reacted by reducing the price (Editorial 2001b).
- Brazil declared it would transfer the technology for ARV production free of charge to all developing countries. There are other efforts under way to export the appropriate technology to produce ARV to poor countries affected by HIV.
- Overall, meanwhile, there are a wide variety of prices for ARV brand and generic drugs. Generic prices are not always lower than the prices for brand-name drugs. Therefore, generics production cannot be the sole option for increasing access to ARV. A mix of different interventions is required, such as voluntary licences, which are given by brand producers to other companies, as was done in South Africa; differential or equity pricing; building manufacturing capacity in poor countries; applying TRIPS safeguards; and re-evaluating and reinterpreting TRIPS regulations.

14.5 Cost-effectiveness

> It is sometimes assumed that HIV prevention is more cost-effective than ARV. This fails to consider that prevention and care must not be separated for an effective fight against AIDS, that the utility of therapy extends far beyond the immediate income gain, and that an increase in the resources of poor countries must also be taken into account.

- A perceived lack of cost-effectiveness of ARV treatment in poor countries has been used as an argument against increasing access to ARV. It is emphasized that HIV prevention is more cost-effective than ARV treatment, so that where resources are scarce, prevention must take priority over treatment. At best a treatment of opportunistic illnesses and palliative care are regarded as cost-effective here (Marseille et al. 2002). However, this approach has encountered increasing criticism.
- Prevention and treatment have synergistic effects which cannot be attained by focusing on prevention alone. It has been demonstrated that prevention without treatment (e.g. voluntary counselling and testing without corresponding medical care) is not credible. Likewise, a strategy purely concentrated on treatment also falls short, because it misses important opportunities to convey prevention options in the care of those

affected by HIV. The "prevention or care" question is thus wrongly posed in this either/or form.
- Prevention and treatment involve different groups of persons. Unequal interventions cannot be compared in a cost-benefit analysis.
- If entire generations die off, there will no longer be anyone left to implement prevention interventions.
- The example of Brazil shows that universal access to ART is a cost-effective intervention for fighting HIV in poorer countries.
- In calculating the cost-effectiveness of ART, in most cases the costs for the therapy were compared with the loss of income which would occur in the event of the premature death of an HIV-infected person. This needs to be reinterpreted, since other costs must be integrated into these calculations besides the immediate loss of income, such as the loss of savings, costs due to orphans, etc. (Commission on Macroeconomics and Health 2001).
- Cost-effectiveness relates to the distribution of limited resources, whereby usually only the resources available to the country in question are integrated into the calculation. However, international discussion about access to ARV focuses precisely on increasing these resources. This can be done by increasing development aid, multilateral financing (e.g. via the Global Fund), debt cancellation, and so on. These measures would strengthen the fight against AIDS either directly or indirectly, via the reduction of poverty.
- In the long term, omitting care will generate costs which will be a great deal higher. However, costs are mostly postponed (i.e. someone other than the originally intended paying party will have to cover the subsequent costs). Among these are the costs generated due to the lack of access to treatment for opportunistic diseases and to life-prolonging ARV treatment, which are borne by families (through their further impoverishment) and society (through the collapse of the social structure). Because these costs do not initially show up (or only covertly) in the budgets of governments and donor organizations, the impression is given that they do not exist.

14.6 Ethics

- It is illegitimate to conduct pure cost-benefit analyses without considering ethical standpoints. Ultimately, there is an ethical obligation to care for people living with HIV/AIDS, such as exists with respect to other diseases. Increasingly, the "right to health" is being recognized. For example, the UN Commission on Human Rights has recognized the right of access to ARV (UN 2001).
- Connected to this is the issue of distributive justice on a global scale. The global responsibility of individuals, states, international communities of states and corporations takes on increasing significance.

> Increasingly, the right to health is acknowledged, which must not be denied to people in poor countries.

14.7 Adherence and treatment literacy

- Adherence to ARV therapy is a measure of how consistently and completely drugs are taken. The argument that poor people would not be able to adhere to ARV drug regimens because of their complexity and a lack of knowledge and skills has often been used to deny access to ARV.
- However, studies have shown that patients in resource-poor settings adhere to ARV drug regimens at levels of more than 90 per cent, which is much more than those in developed nations, where adherence was found to be around 70 per cent (Orrell et al. 2003).
- The people enrolled in these programmes were usually very motivated to take their drugs correctly. In addition, they received special counselling and information on the importance of regular drug use. For example, the South African activist and advocacy movement Treatment Action Campaign engages in "treatment literacy" within communities. It provides information on all aspects related to care and treatment, including knowledge on ARV therapy – the importance of adherence, the medical background, the socio-psychological dimensions, etc.
- In most programmes in poor countries until now, HIV/AIDS education almost exclusively conveyed information about HIV prevention. Treatment options were mentioned only in connection with opportunistic diseases such as tuberculosis. However, in all education programmes it is necessary to discuss every potential treatment, and this includes ARV treatment.

> It is necessary to discuss every treatment option for HIV/AIDS, including ARV treatment.

14.8 Benefits of increased access to ARV

- From the increased access to life-prolonging ARV one can expect advantages for the HIV-infected people themselves, their families and societies as a whole: reduction of AIDS-related deaths and opportunistic infections; lowering of the time and expense for funerals and nursing; reduction in the number of orphans; preservation of the workforce; increase in food security, etc. Thus, one can potentially prevent or alleviate all destructive consequences of the HIV/AIDS epidemic, such as social instability, impoverishment, etc.
- Treatment with ARV can also reduce HIV transmission:
  - Knowledge about the treatability of the illness will increase the willingness to undergo HIV tests.
  - Similarly, as was the case with tuberculosis and leprosy, one can predict that the illness will be demystified through its very treatability.
  - Connected with this, since HIV diagnosis no longer represents a death sentence, HIV-associated stigma will be reduced. Corresponding experiences have already been observed in several pilot projects.
  - Reduction of the viral load in the blood will probably lower infectiousness, and thus also the probability of HIV transmission.
- Until now, ARV drugs in poor countries have often been prescribed and taken in a disorganized way because healthcare workers were inadequately trained and/or the affected persons could not afford a complete

> Increased access to ARV would reduce death rates and HIV-associated illnesses and thus alleviate the economic and social impact of the epidemic. A preventive effect can also be expected, by reducing the stigma and increasing the demand for HIV testing.

therapy. Not taking the drugs according to the standards can result in suboptimal treatment results; moreover, resistances can develop which have negative consequences for the individual patients and (via effects on the course of the HIV epidemic) on population health. To prevent further negative effects through uncontrolled taking of medications, access to ARV has to be increased rapidly. In addition, all those affected, including people active in the healthcare system, must be rapidly informed and trained on all aspects of ARV treatment. The churches have a decisive role to play, since they can reach out to people in communities.

15. HIV/AIDS on the international agenda

15.1 INTERNATIONAL COMMITMENT

- The HIV/AIDS epidemic began slowly at the beginning of the 1980s with rising infection rates among young people and was accompanied by social stigma, fear and a feeling of impotence among many, including those within healthcare systems. For most countries as well as on the international level, AIDS initially represented purely a health problem.
- By 1990, however, many countries had developed national AIDS control programmes, most of which were almost entirely focused on prevention, since treatment was generally ineffective or unaffordable. The epidemic spread more quickly than did the programmes intended to fight it, and in many cases the reaction was not up to the challenge.
- By then, HIV/AIDS was increasingly being perceived as a problem which had its causes in and was reinforced by social and economic inequality, discrimination and marginalization. It was also recognized that the health sector alone could not deal with the problem, and multi-sectorial approaches were to be preferred (Tarantola 2001).
- Nevertheless, the resources made available for fighting HIV/AIDS have remained largely inadequate. The difficulties poor countries face in fighting AIDS effectively rest largely on the fact that they lack the resources to do the job. For example, developing countries often spend more to pay off their foreign debts than they do for the health and education sector. An increase in development aid of just 10 per cent would make €3 billion available annually.
- There has also been a lack of commitment to adequately resource the fight against HIV/AIDS.
- However, there has been some progress in this area and the response to the HIV epidemic has grown more intensive in recent years, on both the national and the international levels.
- In June 2001 the UN held a Special Session of the General Assembly on HIV/AIDS (UNGASS), where the unanimously adopted Declaration committed member states to substantially increase resources for financing the fight against HIV/AIDS on the international level. In addition they set themselves specific goals: 25 per cent reduction of HIV prevalence among young people in the most affected countries by 2005, and globally by 2010; strengthening the protection of human rights for people living with HIV and for vulnerable groups by 2003; treatment and care for HIV-infected people should have the same fundamental importance as prevention; and others (United Nations 2001).
- The UN Security Council has dealt with the theme repeatedly since 2000. Regional and international meetings increasingly have HIV/AIDS on the agenda.
- Despite these developments, commitment to the fight against AIDS on a global scale remains far behind that required. It has been calculated that US$7–10 billion are needed annually to combat AIDS around the world effectively (Schwartlander et al. 2001). There is broad agreement

AIDS has received increasing attention on the international agenda. In June 2001 the UN held a Special Session of the General Assembly on HIV/AIDS, where a far-reaching Declaration of Commitment was adopted.

that such an amount cannot be financed by developing countries, but that it could be easily furnished by the international community. Yet there has not been sufficient political will, particularly in the rich countries, to increase resources to fight AIDS adequately (Attaran and Sachs 2001).

– WHO's Commission on Macroeconomics and Health has calculated that the least-developed countries would have to spend US$30–40 annually per person for health in order to cut by half the premature deaths due to AIDS, malaria and other widespread diseases: this would save the lives of 8 million people per year. However, since this amount far exceeds what these countries can presently pay, the Commission argues that they need long-term support from rich countries. Even with an increase in the health expenditures of the poor countries from US$50 billion to 90 billion by the year 2015, there still remains a financing gap, which must be closed by gradually increasing development aid in the health field from the present figure of around US$3.5 billion to US$29 billion in 2015.

– The financial benefit of this global effort would be many times greater than the investments. The increased productivity and greater economic growth are estimated to be at least US$360 billion per year. Thus, this investment would be highly cost-effective. The Commission demonstrates that such an approach necessitates a rethinking in current development policy (Commission on Macroeconomics and Health 2001).

– Commitment of the affected countries has been stepped up over the past years. In April 2001 at an OAU conference in Abuja, Nigeria, African government heads declared their goal to devote 15 per cent of their budgets for health and the fight against AIDS (Abuja Declaration 2001). Some countries have declared HIV/AIDS a national emergency, and a number of governments and heads of state have publicly declared their willingness to fight HIV/AIDS adequately.

> The difficulties that poor countries face in fighting AIDS effectively rest not least on a lack of resources. US$7–10 billion per year are necessary to fight AIDS globally. However, to a large extent rich countries show a lack of political will to increase resources sufficiently.

> The lives of 8 million people could be saved each year if sufficient resources were provided for fighting the most widespread illnesses in developing countries. The financial benefits alone would be many times greater than the investments.

15.2 GLOBAL FUND TO FIGHT AIDS, TUBERCULOSIS AND MALARIA

– A new instrument on a global level to generate resources is the Global Fund to Fight AIDS, Tuberculosis and Malaria, which was launched at UNGASS in June 2001. These three diseases were identified as creating the biggest burden of disease worldwide, and the Fund was to help finance the fight against them.

– The Global Fund is designed as a financial instrument, not an implementing agency. The most severely affected countries are to receive priority.

– In January 2002 the secretariat and the board started to operate in Geneva. In a unique way the board consists of representatives from developing countries, industrialized countries, NGOs, representatives of affected people, foundations and businesses, and UN organizations as observers. All board members have equal voting rights and no group of countries can make a decision against the will of another group. This is to prevent the domination of recipient countries by donor countries.

– In order to submit a proposal to the Global Fund, countries must form a Country Coordinating Mechanism (CCM). The participation of civil social organizations is obligatory in these CCMs and must be demon-

> Proposals to the Global Fund are submitted through Country Coordinating Mechanisms in which the participation of civil society is obligatory.

strated. Thus far this has functioned satisfactorily to well in quite a few countries, such as Zambia, Haiti, Chile and Sri Lanka.

- Once a CCM has prepared a project proposal it is sent to a Technical Review Panel (TRP) consisting of disease experts both from the North and the South. They look at the technical quality of the proposal, the technical capacity of the applicant to implement the programme and whether the proposal is additional to existing activities.

- The TRP then recommends high quality and viable programmes to the board for approval. This mechanism ensures that there is a participatory and democratic process from the planning stage at the country level, to the TRP and the board. This is quite unique, as there are few if any organizations financing development programmes where recipient countries or representatives have equal decision-making power on all levels to donor countries.

- The Global Fund pursues the policy that countries should purchase drugs at the lowest possible price. This can include both generic and brand-name drugs, depending on the price and patent situation. The only condition is that they must satisfy WHO quality control and they must be procured in a way that respects national and international law.

- By November 2003 the Global Fund had approved US$2.1 billion over two years to 224 programmes in 121 countries and 3 territories, following the review of three proposal rounds in April 2002 and January and October 2003. US$155 million have been disbursed following agreements in 80 per cent of countries with grants.

> The Global Fund has committed US$2.1 billion over two years to 224 programmes in 121 countries.

- Expected outcomes of Global Fund grants over a period of five years include antiretroviral treatment extending to more than 700,000 people living with HIV, tripling current coverage in developing countries; 35 million people reached with voluntary counselling and testing services; and over 1 million orphans supported with medical services, education and community care.

- The Global Fund has achieved a broader local partnership, with non-government representatives constituting 63 per cent of CCM membership and 69 per cent of CCMs, including faith-based organizations (Global Fund 2003).

- The graph shows money spent by the Global Fund by disease (source: Global Fund 2003).

- Through 2004, US$2.9 billion is pledged to the Global Fund, with an additional US$1.9 billion pledged for 2005 to 2008 or for an unspecified period. The overall funding need through 2004 was projected at around US$3.3 billion. The Global Fund is making progress in resource mobilization.

- There remain some questions which require further clarification: how can the long-term financial funding of the Global Fund be assured, and how can donor governments be prevented from redirecting resources for the Fund from other areas? The Ecumenical Advocacy Alliance also supports the Global Fund, and is fighting for it to be adequately funded with financial resources specially allocated for this purpose (Ecumenical Advocacy Alliance 2001).

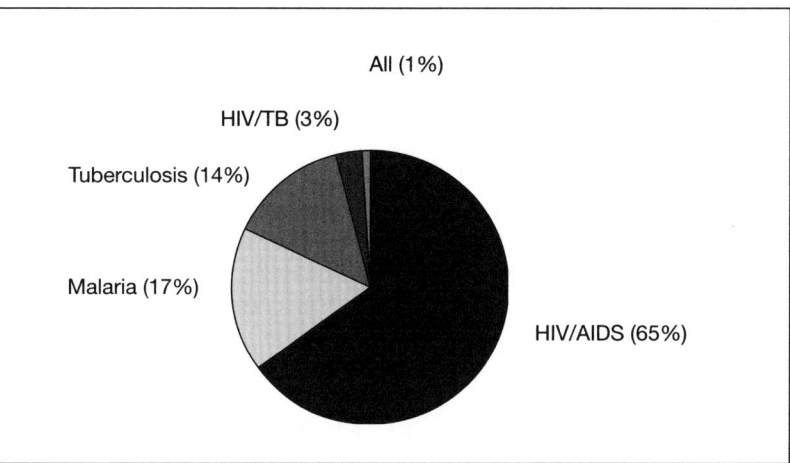

- For all these open questions, the Global Fund represents an innovative and, despite all the risks, promising approach for changing the worldwide inequality in healthcare between rich and poor countries. The potential can be realized if, through prudent decision-making and management of resources, the Global Fund finds broad acceptance in the future.

16. Advocacy and lobbying

Advocacy acts on behalf of people who are affected by HIV/AIDS: among the public and among decision-makers in politics, churches and the private sector. It played an essential role in getting the topic of HIV/AIDS onto the international agenda.

- Advocacy has acquired increasing importance in the fight against HIV/AIDS. Advocacy and lobbying work attempts to influence the governments of affected countries, to put HIV/AIDS on the political agenda, and to secure the necessary allocation of resources for fighting AIDS.
- On the global level, a series of organizations from civil society, such as Médecins sans Frontières, have for years undertaken advocacy work for the human rights of those affected by HIV, for increased access to treatment, and so on.
- In September 2002 a new coalition of the most wide-ranging organizations from civil society, the UN, governments, foundations, the private sector, etc. was constituted under the name International Treatment Access Coalition (ITAC). Its objective is to increase access to HIV treatment for all people who need it (International Treatment Access Coalition 2002).

The AIDS activist movement Treatment Action Campaign in South Africa exemplifies successful lobbying and advocacy.

- In South Africa, the Treatment Action Campaign (TAC), which was founded in 1998, performs advocacy and lobbying work as well as legal interventions: it contributed to the withdrawal of the lawsuit of multinational pharmaceutical companies; it successfully sued the government in order to demand a programme for reducing mother-to-child transmission of HIV; it lobbied for a National Treatment Plan; and filed lawsuits against two pharmaceutical companies (GlaxoSmithKline and Boehringer Ingelheim) for overpricing their ARV drugs in South Africa (TAC 2003).
- In August 2002, PATAM (the Pan African Treatment Access Movement) was founded to do advocacy and lobbying on national levels in Africa for increased access to ARV.
- International advocacy and lobbying played an essential role in putting HIV/AIDS on the international agenda and prompted stronger discussions of global responsibility in this context.
- The churches and their agencies have a special responsibility here, since as social forces and power factors they can exert a far-reaching influence. Advocacy should also take place within church structures. Target groups of advocacy include the executive level and staff in organizations, church communities and people outside those communities.
- Inspired by the Ecumenical Advocacy Alliance, Action against AIDS was founded in Germany as a campaign that wishes to mobilize the German public and put pressure on national and international political decision-makers in order to attain the allocation of greater resources for fighting AIDS. Over 40 organizations and churches have become members of the campaign, and over 1,000 grassroots groups are registered as supporters.
- Ecumenical Advocacy Alliance: see p. 99.

17. Culture and tradition

17.1 BIOMEDICAL, RELIGIOUS AND TRADITIONAL FRAMEWORK

- After more than 20 years of a devastating HIV/AIDS pandemic there remain some very fundamental questions: why have not more countries been able to prevent this disease spiral out of control when the main concepts of prevention and care have been known for many years? Why have not more people adopted safer sex behaviour despite being well informed about the main ways of transmission and the best protective measures? To answer these questions one has to consider the cultural perception of disease, its cause and effect, as well as the cultural context of sexuality – with all its moral connotations and consequences.

- Of course, it has to be emphasized that one cannot speak of the African, European or Asian culture. Traditions and cultural frameworks usually relate only to specific ethnic groups or geographical regions sharing historical developments and philosophical backgrounds. Nevertheless, there appear to be certain paradigms or discourses that might help to explain the specific problems posed by HIV/AIDS.

- Anthropological research has increasingly differentiated between at least three different frameworks or discourses which are of great importance for the interpretation of HIV/AIDS: the biomedical, the religious and the traditional.

> The biomedical, the religious and the traditional framework are three important discourses in the interpretation of HIV/AIDS.

- From research in his native country of Zambia, C. Bawa Yamba, an anthropologist who did extensive studies on AIDS, concludes: "Rural Africans now find themselves the target of three competing and contradictory discourses about responsibility, each of which claims to tell them how to lead safe lives free from AIDS. The first, represented by the biomedical paradigm, professes sure knowledge about the aetiology and epidemiology of HIV/AIDS but is unable to cure it; the second, the missionary discourse, preaches abstinence and encourages a revival of traditional beliefs and rules of morality as the only way to manage and survive AIDS; while the third is the traditional discourse – represented by traditional healers and witch finders – which professes sure knowledge and the ability to eradicate evil" (Yamba 1997).

- Different societies, cultures and social contexts attach varying importance to these three paradigms. In relation to HIV/AIDS, all of them contribute to explanations and interpretations that strongly influence the behaviour of people (Benn 2002a).

- The biomedical or scientific framework has strongly influenced developments in technology, medicine and other areas that have become part of our daily life. It understands the processes of nature as phenomena following certain rules that are not influenced by any metaphysical powers. Instead, many processes are governed by chance and outcomes can only be calculated as probabilities using statistical methods.

> The biomedical framework understands the processes of nature as phenomena following certain rules that are not influenced by any metaphysical powers.

- Scientists break down very complex organisms or processes into small units and observe the influence of defined interventions in comparison to processes that have not been altered. This has led to great breakthroughs in many areas. It is the basis for scientific clinical research on diseases and therapies. These methods have helped to identify the virus that causes AIDS, find tests that can prove its presence in human beings and develop drugs that can at least prevent the multiplication of the virus in the human body.

– These methods can also be applied to public health interventions examining the health of groups of people or whole populations. Thus, to assess a certain method in AIDS prevention (e.g. sex education, condom promotion or treatment of STIs), one compares a population that received a specific intervention with a population that did not, excluding other factors that might explain any differences.

– However, research that follows the scientific paradigm finds it very difficult to take into account factors like cultural perceptions, particularly if they do not fit into the worldview of the researcher.

– The religious framework is shaped by a worldview developed over a long period of time in the major world religions. Many of the regions that are most severely hit by HIV/AIDS are deeply influenced by both Christianity and Islam. These two religions have been introduced in Africa, Latin America and large parts of Asia by missionaries, traders and conquerors and usually exist alongside more traditional religious practices. They have brought distinct interpretations of disease and healing.

> The religious framework is based on the assumption that there is a God who influences both creation and history and who is accessible through prayer and devotion.

– Despite the great variety of different interpretations of theological issues in various denominations and religious traditions, the central element of the religious framework is based on the assumption that there is a God who influences both creation and history and who is accessible through prayer and devotion. This has consequences for the religious understanding of the origin of AIDS. It also invokes, as in all religions, a code of moral norms directly impacting upon any understanding of a disease related to human behaviour.

– Religious norms regarding human sexuality are surprisingly similar. Muslims, Jews, Christians and other religions largely adhere to the ideal of sexuality as having its rightful place in lifelong marriage. Strict norms about pre-marital abstinence and faithfulness in marriage arise. Variation comes in the consequences of this ideal for teaching, pastoral counselling and advice for those who cannot follow the ideal (World Council of Churches 2001).

> The traditional framework is influenced by religion, but in a form that is more related to local beliefs and traditions.

– A traditional framework is defined as a worldview that is also strongly influenced by religion, but in a form that is more related to local beliefs and traditions. In this context negative events such as diseases or untimely death are often interpreted as being caused by evil forces or spirits.

– It has to be acknowledged that within the traditional framework there is a multitude of explanations for disease. Some of them differentiate between natural and supernatural causes and the concept of infectious agents (worms, tiny insects) is quite prominent in some cultures (Green 1999).

– However, HIV/AIDS in particular, as a new and in many ways mysterious disease affecting mainly young people not expected to die of natural causes, is frequently explained by a curse inflicted upon somebody after transgression of taboos and/or by witchcraft. "Witchcraft" might have a purely negative connotation in Western cultures, but it can be a very natural and relevant interpretation in many societies. It can simply mean that someone or something is responsible for this evil and that the identification of the source of evil is a precondition for finding a cure or solution.

– Unfortunately in the case of HIV/AIDS this traditional interpretation of witchcraft as a legitimate explanation might also lead to a strategy of avoidance, thus inhibiting any efforts to influence individual behaviour.

– The question of whether to promote or reject the use of latex condoms can illustrate the argument about the importance of these three different frameworks. For the scientific community, condoms have been the mainstay of recommended public health intervention since the beginning of the epidemic. Scientists argue that if two persons have sexual intercourse and one person is already HIV-infected and they use a condom correctly, the risk for the non-infected partner is almost negligible. Although condoms are not an absolute protection against HIV transmission, for scientists working in the scientific framework of statistical analysis and the comparison of relative risks the answer is still very convincing: condoms are highly effective in the prevention of HIV.

> For example, the three paradigms look differently at the use of condoms in HIV prevention.

– For religious leaders, not used to thinking in statistical terms but in absolute truths, the answer might also be clear: condoms are not 100 per cent effective, therefore they cannot be the solution. Such leaders are afraid that the promotion of condoms might undermine their proclaimed ideal of abstinence before and faithfulness during marriage. Any further argument will then depend on whether a particular church tradition or leadership will accept the reality that extra-marital relationships do occur, and that negative consequences in the form of disease can be prevented, or whether they feel that this acknowledgement diminishes the force of their argument.

– The official study of the World Council of Churches (WCC) on HIV/AIDS adopted by the Central Committee in 1996 tried to keep the balance between empirical evidence for the effectiveness of condoms and concerns about promiscuous behaviour: "Without blessing or encouraging promiscuity, we recognize the reality of human sexual relationships and practice and the existence of HIV in the world. Scientific evidence has demonstrated that education on positive measures of prevention and the provision and use of condoms help to prevent transmission of the virus and the consequent suffering and death for many of those infected. Should not the churches, in the light of these facts, recognize the use of condoms as a method of prevention of HIV?" (WCC 1997).

– In spite of this statement many churches, even those who are members of the WCC, are still reluctant to endorse publicly the use of condoms to prevent HIV, possibly because for them the dilemma between ideal and reality is still not resolved.

– For the traditional framework, there is probably a very different line of argument. If the disease is believed to be caused by witchcraft and evil forces then, of course, the use of condoms cannot be a viable defence against these forces unless condoms are perceived as having magical powers. The idea of personal responsibility does not help either, because the crucial forces are usually outside the control of any individual, who would feel rather helpless on their own against this overwhelming threat.

17.2 INTEGRATION OF THE PARADIGMS

- If progress is to be achieved in the future the three paradigms cannot remain in contradiction to each other because that would be counter-productive for any preventive efforts. The first step should be that each person engaged in a serious discourse about HIV/AIDS should understand that there is more than one legitimate way to interpret disease and the best ways to address it. A fruitful dialogue and as far as possible the integration of paradigms into useful frameworks could help lead us out of the current situation with different explanations contradicting each other.
- There are a number of examples of the integration of different paradigms:
  - In Uganda young people have changed their sexual behaviour, which is partially due to the integration of medical-scientific explanations of HIV transmission into their own cultural frameworks.
  - In Zambia, the traditional practice of widow cleansing through sexual intercourse is increasingly being replaced by other more symbolic practices entailing no risk of HIV infection. People have retained the positive values of traditional practices like social support for widows, while accepting scientific explanations about the risk of HIV transmission.
  - In Tanzania traditional healers have used the method of scarification with razor blades or other sharp instruments for their treatment. This method carried a risk of transmitting HIV from one person to the other because instruments were not sterilized between use. After education seminars the practice was changed and patients were asked to bring their own razor blades. Without abandoning the practice altogether its dangerous aspects were avoided.
- Access to effective treatment can also contribute to the integration of paradigms. People tend to believe messages that are consistent and make sense. The scientific explanation about the transmission of malaria parasites via mosquitoes is easier to accept if there are also drugs to cure the fever. Personal experience will reinforce the scientific explanation. The same applies to many other treatable diseases, like tuberculosis or diarrhoea. Treatment for HIV/AIDS will ultimately reduce the mystery surrounding this disease and reinforce preventive messages.
- None of the frameworks described here is cast in stone and so rigid that it cannot be changed or adapted. Culture is a dynamic process – this also applies to the traditional framework. The primary goal of all paradigms is to preserve life and to provide explanations for people to help them cope with the various challenges of life.
- One increasingly hears from churches a call to question culture critically and to confront religious content and its interplay with tradition. In so

doing, culture is never simply to be rejected. It is precisely the churches who emphasize that the positive aspect in culture and tradition must be preserved and promoted, but that the harmful practices which limit and destroy people must be challenged and – if necessary – changed. Thus the HIV epidemic, with all its catastrophic consequences, can prompt a critical confrontation with existing paradigms and lead to an improvement in the lives of human beings (Ecumenical Consultation 2001).

18. Churches, theology and HIV/AIDS

18.1 CHURCHES AND AIDS

Churches have often had significant difficulties in dealing constructively with HIV/AIDS, and at times they have done more to impede rather than facilitate effective prevention efforts. In many countries, however, the churches have made an essential contribution to effective education and to humane treatment of people with HIV/AIDS.

- AIDS and the churches is a complex theme. For many, the churches are more part of the problem than of the solution. They are associated with rigid sexual morality and the rejection of preventive measures. Particularly sensitive issues are sex education for young people, the use of condoms, and gender roles.

- The churches have indeed often had significant difficulties in dealing constructively with the topic of HIV/AIDS, and often they have done more to impede than facilitate effective prevention efforts. This has also been publicly acknowledged and regretted. Thus, the study of the World Council of Churches on HIV/AIDS states: "the reaction of the churches has by and large been inadequate, and in some cases has made the problem even worse" (WCC 1997).

- However, this statement expresses only a part of the reality. In many countries, the churches have made a definite contribution to effective education and humane care for people with HIV/AIDS.

- Not only individual churches, but also ecumenical institutions have made a commitment to the fight against AIDS. As early as 1987 the executive committee of the WCC issued a prophetic statement: "The AIDS crisis challenges us profoundly to be the church in deed and in truth: to be the church as a healing community" (WCC 1987).

- Since then the churches have not only engaged in intensive theological debate but also started many different initiatives.

- Churches also are encouraged to look at how they are dealing with people living with HIV within their communities, among clergy, etc. The Action Plan of the Ecumenical Consultation of the Churches in Africa on HIV/AIDS demands that people with HIV should have a firm place in the churches, where they are safe and know that they are accepted (Ecumenical Consultation 2001).

- The churches have a responsibility to encourage their members and to support them in openly declaring their positive HIV status. They should also create a safe space for HIV-positive clergy. Canon Gideon Byamugisha, one of the first clergy to declare openly their positive HIV status, has been on the forefront of living openly with HIV within the church for 10 years. In commemoration of his living openly with HIV, in September 2003 the African Network of Religious Leaders Living with or Affected by HIV/AIDS (ANERELA+) was founded. Its vision is "to have a religion where religious leaders living positively and affected by HIV/AIDS are empowered to live openly as witnesses to hope and be forces for change in their communities". ANERELA+ can be contacted under: limpopo@global.co.za.

18.2 ACTIVITIES AND INITIATIVES

18.2.1 Ecumenical Advocacy Alliance

– The Ecumenical Advocacy Alliance was founded in 2000 and embraces more than 60 churches and church organizations throughout the world, including the World Council of Churches and the Lutheran World Federation. The EAA is an ecumenical network for international cooperation in advocacy: it wishes to "strengthen the ecumenical witness in important social, political and economic issues" (Ecumenical Advocacy Alliance 2001a).

– The Alliance has selected HIV/AIDS as a priority issue alongside global trade. Thus, AIDS worldwide should become a primary topic of the advocacy of churches, church related development agencies and the ecumenical family. With the Action Plan for 2002–2004, the HIV/AIDS Campaign of the Ecumenical Advocacy Alliance wishes to achieve the following goals:

- Deploy the churches on behalf of the rights and dignity of people living with HIV and to fight discrimination and stigmatization.
- Promote prevention which combats the roots of people's vulnerability to HIV infection.
- Mobilize resources for prevention, care and treatment.
- Increase access to care and treatment.

> The Ecumenical Advocacy Alliance has set as its objective making HIV/AIDS throughout the world a primary topic of advocacy on the part of the churches, church development agencies and the ecumenical family.

18.2.2 Ecumenical HIV/AIDS Initiative in Africa

– In 2001, consultations of church representatives were held in Eastern, Western and Southern Africa, and in November of the same year a conference with over 100 church representatives took place in Nairobi, Kenya. The Ecumenical Consultation of the Churches in Africa on HIV/AIDS adopted a far-reaching Action Plan (Ecumenical Consultation 2001).

> In November 2001 an Ecumenical Consultation on HIV/AIDS was held in Nairobi.

– Since April 2002 the Ecumenical HIV/AIDS Initiative in Africa has been operational. A central coordinator and four regional coordinators for Eastern, Southern, Western and Central Africa are networking activities in their respective regions and provide information on existing programmes and projects of the churches and religious organizations. The Initiative also supported the production of theological materials on HIV/AIDS, to be used in sermons, theological training, communities, etc. Its reports and publications can be found under http://www.wcc-coe.org/wcc/what/mission/ehaia-index.html. They can be contacted under cma@wcc-coe.org.

> The Ecumenical HIV/AIDS Initiative has been establishing information and action networks on HIV/AIDS among the churches in Africa.

18.2.3 South Asia Ecumenical Partnership Programme

– The Christian Conference in Asia (CCA) published a declaration on HIV/AIDS (CCA 2001) and together with the WCC in July 2002 in Colombo organized an HIV/AIDS Consultation of the Southern Asian churches. Its report regards HIV prevention and fighting HIV-associated stigma in South Asia as urgent missions for the churches.

- The South Asia Ecumenical Partnership Programme has been established since then. It has as one of its priority areas HIV/AIDS and also aims at mainstreaming HIV/AIDS into its other programme components (SAEPP 2003). Information to be found under http://www.wcc-coe.org/wcc/what/regional/saepp-guidelines.pdf.
- Further initiatives of this kind are under way.

18.2.4 Ecumenical Pharmaceutical Network

- Developing out of the Pharmaceutical Programme under the WCC, the Ecumenical Pharmaceutical Network evolved with the goal to support healthcare providers, at all levels, in their efforts to improve patient care through proper drug management and use, especially (but not exclusively) in church-related health institutions and programmes. Specifically, the Network works towards ensuring that effective and appropriate Essential Drug Concepts and Rational Drug Use policies are implemented in church related health facilities and programmes.
- The Ecumenical Pharmaceutical Network has developed an inventory of health institutions that provide ARV treatment and the number of people trained in management of ARV treatment in Africa. Information can be found under http://www.epnetwork.org/. It can be contacted under epn@wanachi.com.

18.3 Responsibilities, successes and potentials

> Churches bear a special responsibility in the fight against AIDS, because such action can be derived from their mission of salvation entrusted to them by Jesus Christ.

> Churches' social and medical institutions allow them to make a direct contribution to fighting AIDS. Moreover, churches have a wide range of resources and a network which reaches many people.

- There is increasing hope that churches will become active partners in fighting HIV/AIDS and thus fulfil their true calling. For several reasons the churches bear a special responsibility with regard to HIV/AIDS:
  - The message and the actions of Jesus were aimed at bringing people comprehensive salvation, as well as integrating victims of discrimination and social and religious outcasts. This mission also applies for the followers of Jesus in the various churches.
  - Churches are part of civil society. They cannot and must not ignore the burning social problems around them, but rather are called upon to make their contribution to resolving these problems.
  - Churches maintain important social and medical institutions which can make a direct contribution to fighting HIV/AIDS.
  - Churches claim to have an impact on the behaviour of people. The objective is to impart values and ethical standards which are life-enhancing and life-preserving. Especially with an essentially sexually transmitted disease such as HIV/AIDS, the churches are called upon to have a responsible impact on behaviours and social conditions so that the risk of infection can be reduced.
  - Churches have a pastoral mission to practise solidarity with all people who, directly or indirectly, suffer from HIV/AIDS and offer them spiritual as well as material assistance.
  - In many parts of the world, the churches hold an extraordinary significance for individuals and communities. In Africa, Asia and Latin

America, churches play a role in the life of people which is quite different from their role in more secularized countries.

- Faith-based organizations have contributed decisively to preventing the spread of HIV in Senegal, and to rolling back the epidemic in Uganda (Green 2003). This makes clear the importance of the churches, which extends far beyond the relevance for their "members" to fulfil an important socio-political mission.

- For example, in a study in South Africa, those surveyed indicated that religious organizations were for them an important source of information on HIV/AIDS (HSRC 2002).

> In principle, all areas in the fight against AIDS can be dealt with by the churches: education, care in health facilities and communities, addressing marginal and vulnerable groups, advocacy and lobbying.

- In education, information and instruction, churches can reach many people, above all young people, women, etc.

- In some cases churches can also reach marginalized population groups, such as indigenous people, CSWs, drug addicts and street children. Although some churches may have reservations about these marginal groups, there are very often committed Christians working in areas that are difficult to access for other organizations.

- Churches are also active in countries and situations where the political structure is threatened or lacking altogether, such as in conditions of war and civil unrest, where church structures and resources can be among the few institutions which have access to the people and are in a position to operate across dividing lines.

- The church agencies and their partners can contribute to changing policies through lobbying work and advocacy with the governments in both North and South and with international institutions.

- Churches and their organizations also have an important task in the area of care for those affected by HIV:

  - In several countries there exist home care projects, programmes for the care of orphans and so on, within the churches or sponsored by secular organizations. There is a need for greater expansion of these interventions and support for the existing initiatives.

  - In many countries throughout the world the churches are important healthcare providers. In Kenya, for example, churches run about 40 per cent of all hospital services, and in Zimbabwe the corresponding figure is 68 per cent. Church hospitals are often better equipped than government institutions, and can therefore offer more effective and better-quality care. AIDS has given a special urgency to discussions of the support of these healthcare institutions by development agencies. This also includes the area of antiretroviral therapy.

> Church health facilities have a decisive role in connection with AIDS.

- Many projects are successful on a small scale (e.g. on the community level) but the necessary resources are lacking to implement them on a large scale. Churches should coordinate their efforts and expand individual projects which have proven successful and implement them on a larger scale (scaling up). These can be pilot projects which, for example, identify new dimensions in the fight against AIDS and their practicability. These projects then serve as Best Practices (i.e. as models from which other stakeholders can learn).

> Churches can implement pilot projects which, due to their model-like character, can serve as Best Practices.

- Churches have a wide range of resources. They have networks which extend into the most remote areas of countries. The most important resource are the faithful, the members of the church themselves, with their various gifts and talents, many of whom offer their work to the church communities as volunteers (Greyling 2001).
- Churches are also increasingly being perceived internationally and by secular organizations as important partners in overcoming AIDS. Organizations like the World Health Organization, UNAIDS and the Global Fund to Fight AIDS, Tuberculosis and Malaria look to the churches as true partners who can help to achieve ambitious objectives in international health through their extensive experience and infrastructure in the provision of healthcare.
- Churches and religious groups are especially well suited for providing spiritual care to those affected by HIV. This dimension is often undervalued in more secular discussions. In many cases, people who had turned away from their faith find their way back to the church and to God. Beyond this, many people have a strong belief in the power of divine providence and love. This faith places the concern for their own fate and that of the family in the hands of God.
- However, good spiritual care also depends on an appropriate theology which does not condemn those who are affected and which conveys an image of the church as the body of Christ, from which no one may be excluded on the basis of a disease.

> *Churches are well suited for providing spiritual care to those affected by HIV. This dimension is often undervalued in more secular discussions.*

18.4 Theological aspects

- HIV/AIDS touches on a number of important theological issues: the role of disease in God's creation, the understanding of suffering and death, the interpretation of sin and forgiveness, love and acceptance, the concept of sexuality and gender relations. The perennial question of what constitutes the church and how the followers of Christ build truly healing communities has enormous consequences in the context of HIV/AIDS.
- Many theologians and churches have done seminal work on these questions. One study that has particular relevance in the ecumenical movement and that has inspired many of the activities cited above is recommended for further study. In 1994 the WCC commissioned a consultative group to prepare a study on the theological, ethical and social issues relating to HIV/AIDS. The study was officially adopted by the Central Committee of the WCC in 1996 and recommended to all member churches for further study and implementation. The document was published by WCC publications in 1997 with the title "Facing AIDS: The challenge, the churches' response". Some of the most important findings will be presented here, as they can stimulate further discussion and theological research.

> *The WCC published "Facing AIDS" in 1997, which was recommended to all member churches for further study and implementation.*

18.4.1 Acceptance and stigma

- God, in Jesus Christ, is particularly near to the disadvantaged, oppressed and outcasts. In many societies this includes people living with

HIV/AIDS. If Christians deny community to these people, not only do they violate human rights, but they also deny the community and solidarity which God offers to all human beings.

- "When people and churches live out of relationship with God and follow Jesus, therefore, they will be continually open to others and offer relationship to them, even to those who seem very different. Just as there is no closing off of relationships in the gospel accounts of Jesus, so churches cannot withdraw into being congenial groups of the like-minded, refusing openness to and esteem for others who are physically or socially different" (WCC 1997: 23).

- "In a community of care, acceptance moves from a simple avoidance of being judgmental to an embracing of who we are individually and, more importantly, together – the difference between receiving someone into your home as a guest, who remains "other", and embracing someone as a rightful member of the family. The presence of HIV in our community – particularly, but not exclusively, in the church community – requires this shift in our understanding of acceptance. We are not called simply to offer charity to those whose physical bodies have the virus. Our undeniable belonging to the community challenges us to embrace the fact, however painful, that the virus has come into our body" (WCC 1997: 29).

- "The church, by its very nature as the body of Christ, calls its members to become healing communities. Despite the extent and complexity of the problems raised by HIV/AIDS, the churches can make an effective healing witness towards those affected. The experience of love, acceptance and support within a community where God's love is made manifest can be a powerful healing force. This means that the church should not – as was often the case when AIDS was first recognized in the gay community – exclude, stigmatize and blame persons on the basis of behaviour which many local congregations and churches judge to be unacceptable" (WCC 1997: 77).

> The church, by its very nature as the body of Christ, calls its members to become healing communities.

18.4.2 Sexuality

- The study "Facing AIDS" promotes a comprehensive understanding of sexuality unconstrained to its erotic aspect, although affirming it. Sexuality is a gift from God which can bring great happiness and fulfilment. At the same time, sexual intimacy is also a moment of particular vulnerability.

> Sexuality is a gift from God and an integral part of human identity.

- "Sexuality is an integral part of human identity. It is expressed in a variety of ways, but finds particular expression in intimate human relationship. It is 'erotic' in the classical sense, that is, it drives one to move beyond oneself into encounter with another in a relationship. And while this aspect of human identity finds particular expression in the dimension of physical intimacy, it cannot be separated from its emotional, intellectual, spiritual and social dimensions. A Christian understanding of sexuality seeks to take account of the fullness of all these dimensions, yet recognizes the mystery which God has given to human beings in sexuality as a whole" (WCC 1977:30).

- "Along with its potential for bringing the richness of intimacy and joy to human relationships, sexuality makes people particularly vulnerable

> Sexuality makes people particularly vulnerable – to each other and to social forces.

– to each other and to social forces. In connection with HIV/AIDS, sexuality increases vulnerability in two ways. First of all, many physical expressions of sexuality can bring one into contact with HIV infection. Second, the very fact that humans are sexual beings makes them vulnerable to the many and varied social factors which influence moral decisions and actions" (WCC 1997: 31).

- The WCC study had no mandate to look at the issue of homosexuality, which continues to be a very divisive topic in many churches. But the study group was at least able to acknowledge the important role the gay community has played in care and prevention and to emphasize the need for further collaboration and mutual understanding. Unfortunately, it fell short of apologizing for the stigma and discrimination of homosexual people to which the churches undoubtedly have contributed.

- "Gay men, who were among the first to be affected by the pandemic and often play a very significant role in care and prevention, have frequently been condemned and marginalized by the churches. Both parties must enter into a new relationship to make for more effective prevention and mutual care" (WCC 1997: 33).

18.4.3 The church as the body of Christ

- The WCC study uses the image of the church as the body of Christ. Particularly important is the understanding of the church as an inclusive community which should not separate itself and ostracize people, but be transparent for the love offered in Jesus Christ. It should be a healing community facilitating openness and the experience of fullness of life for all its members.

- "As the body of Christ, the church is to be the place where God's healing love is experienced and shown forth and God's promise of abundant life is made freely available. Because all persons fall within the scope of God's love and are honoured with Christ's care, we are called to honour one another as if in each person we encounter Christ himself" (WCC 1997: 43).

- "As Christ identifies with our suffering and enters into it, so the church as the body of Christ is called to enter into the suffering of others, to stand with them against all rejection and despair. This is not an option; it is the church's vocation. And because it is the body of Christ – who died for all and who enters into the suffering of all – the church cannot exclude anyone who needs Christ, certainly not those living with HIV/AIDS" (WCC 1977:44).

- "In opening itself to persons living with HIV/AIDS, in entering into their suffering and bearing it with them, in standing with them against rejection and despair, the churches express more fully what it is to be the body of Christ. And as the church enters into solidarity with persons living with HIV/AIDS, its hope in God's promise of abundant life comes alive and becomes visible to the world" (WCC 1997: 44).

- Despite a great deal of theological groundwork, including the WCC study, many churches still find it difficult to accept people with HIV/AIDS without prejudice, and to promote and support all education

> Despite a great deal of theological groundwork, many churches still find it difficult to accept people with HIV/AIDS without prejudice. A theology that fully accepts PLWHA has to be included in theological training.

and prevention efforts. Clearly, more work is needed within church denominations and on an ecumenical, interdenominational basis.
- Finally, it is extremely important that theological studies be implemented on a local, congregational level. For this to happen it has to be included systematically in theological education in seminaries and universities. Efforts in this direction are under way, some of them supported by the Ecumenical HIV/AIDS Initiative in Africa.

19. Mainstreaming HIV/AIDS

19.1 What is mainstreaming HIV/AIDS?

> Mainstreaming HIV/AIDS means that the topic HIV/AIDS becomes part of the "mainstream" of organizations: it should not be treated as one topic among many but rather as a cross-cutting issue that has to be dealt with at all levels within organizations.

– All stakeholders engaged in development work should contribute to the fight against HIV/AIDS through prevention, care and impact mitigation. "Mainstreaming HIV/AIDS" is an important means to achieve this goal, as it ensures that HIV/AIDS is adequately addressed by organizations and programmes. The topic of HIV/AIDS should become part of the "mainstream" of organizations: it should not be treated as one topic among many but rather as a cross-cutting issue that has to be dealt with at all levels and aspects within organizations, programmes and projects.

– Solutions to the challenges may vary according to context. In any case, they have to be identified by the various organizations and programmes themselves. In this way, mainstreaming HIV/AIDS is a process and will itself be a tool to enhance awareness of HIV/AIDS and contribute to fighting it effectively.

– Organizations may be hesitant to undertake the mainstreaming HIV/AIDS because they assume that it requires additional resources. However, mainstreaming is not a matter of securing additional funds and initiating new, separate projects specifically designed to address HIV/AIDS. Mainstreaming HIV/AIDS should be an objective for all organizations in development work: for AIDS organizations and programmes (programmes that specifically and explicitly address HIV/AIDS) and for all other organizations and programmes (for example, rural development, income generation, gender programmes, peace and conflict, etc.).

> Mainstreaming does not imply that all organizations should become "AIDS organizations" and/or develop fully-fledged AIDS programmes. They should continue with the focus they already have. It may, however, be necessary to include some new activities.

– Mainstreaming does not imply that all organizations should become "AIDS organizations" and/or develop fully-fledged AIDS programmes. They should continue with the focus they already have. It may, however, be necessary to include some new activities.

– In this process, existing expertise can be utilized (e.g. using resource persons/experts from other organizations to provide training). A wealth of experiences and best practices on HIV/AIDS already exists among organizations and programmes and can be shared. Networking with other organizations should be established and/or strengthened (e.g. referring beneficiaries and staff to counselling services).

– Mainstreaming should, however, also be undertaken by AIDS programmes. Although these organizations focus their activities on HIV prevention and care, there is likely to be a need for mainstreaming activities, for example to design an HIV/AIDS policy.

– Mainstreaming HIV/AIDS should promote gender equity. The challenging of gender roles, the consideration of women's needs and the sensitization of men to their responsibilities to promote gender equity should be taken into account in all activities concerning the mainstreaming of HIV/AIDS.

– At present, the need to address HIV/AIDS may not appear to be so urgent for many organizations in Asia and other parts of the globe where the epidemic's impact may not have been felt so drastically as elsewhere, and where other social and political problems may seem more pressing. However, there is no place on earth that does not face the threat of the epidemic developing into a crisis, with many countries already well on their way down this path. The discussion of what mainstreaming entails in different epidemiological and social contexts continues, and organizations can define the mainstreaming of HIV/AIDS so it is appropriate to their local circumstances.

19.2 ORGANIZATIONAL LEVEL

- What does mainstreaming HIV/AIDS entail at the organizational level, within an organization/programme itself? At this level, organizations can address the breaking of the silence on HIV/AIDS, reducing stigmatization, developing an AIDS policy, taking care of people infected with and affected by HIV among staff and volunteers, and other issues.
- HIV should be acknowledged as an issue that is of concern to all. This also involves some engagement on a more personal level. People should realize that "business as usual" will not suffice to contain the spread of HIV.
- The silence around AIDS enhances stigmatization and is an obstacle to HIV prevention. It is therefore important for organizations, programmes and projects to address and discuss all matters regarding HIV/AIDS openly, including HIV prevention, epidemiology, care and treatment options, vulnerability to HIV infection, social and economic impact, and gender equity. Discussions and awareness raising on HIV/AIDS can be undertaken at meetings, workshops, etc. They have to include all departments, hierarchy levels, staff and volunteers. Taboo issues, such as homosexuality, drug abuse, sex work, sexual violence, and their interdependence with HIV/AIDS, should be addressed.
- Although information on HIV/AIDS has already been provided for some years, there is still a need for education and information on HIV/AIDS. Messages need to be repeated and to be voiced in different contexts and settings, such as the workplace.
- Capacity building among programme staff and volunteers should be done to empower them to address HIV/AIDS adequately. This can be done through training, for example in counselling skills, spiritual care, home-based care and other areas.
- Churches have a special responsibility, since they are influential as role models and decision makers within communities and in society at large. Churches should openly address HIV/AIDS in all activities and at all levels: among church leadership, clergy, laity and communities.
- In sub-Saharan Africa, all organizations and programmes are affected by the social and economic impact of AIDS. An HIV/AIDS policy can assist an organization to cope with the impact of the HIV epidemic on its capacity. This impact can be felt through the working hours lost due to chronic sickness of staff and volunteers; following premature deaths, posts will either be vacant or may be filled with less trained people; the subsequent high staff turnover and/or drop out rate often lead to decreas-

> At an organizational level, mainstreaming can address the breaking of the silence on HIV/AIDS, reducing stigmatization, developing an AIDS policy, taking care of people infected and affected by HIV among staff and volunteers, and other issues.

> An HIV/AIDS policy can assist organizations to cope with the impact of the HIV epidemic on their capacity.

ing performance within the organization; staff and volunteers are often absent from work because they care for the chronically sick at home (particularly female staff) and attend funerals; through the loss of a breadwinner, families of staff and volunteers may become impoverished; many families care for orphans, widows and other people affected by HIV. These factors place huge strains on families that also affect the organizations where these people work.

– An HIV/AIDS policy should also consider how to provide comprehensive care for staff and volunteers living with and affected by HIV (i.e. medical treatment, including access to antiretroviral therapy, and social and spiritual support). Organizations do not have to provide the whole range of care options themselves, yet access to care and treatment should be facilitated as far as possible through networking with other organizations and the referral of people in need.

– Organizations and programmes must not discriminate against persons infected with and affected by HIV. In particular, policies should ensure that HIV-infected persons do not lose their jobs because of their HIV status; HIV testing must not be a condition for hiring and/or continuation of employment; people living with HIV/AIDS should not be discriminated against or stigmatized in any way at their place of work.

> Organizations and programmes must not discriminate against people infected with and affected by HIV.

– Not to discriminate against PLWHA is a matter of organizations' credibility in the fight against AIDS. Since all HIV interventions should aim at reducing the stigma and embracing PLWHA into communities, programme policies and practices should reflect these principles, and organizations should adhere to them in regard to their own staff and volunteers.

19.3 PROGRAMME IMPLEMENTATION LEVEL

– Mainstreaming HIV/AIDS should also deal with
  • the impact of the HIV/AIDS epidemic on programme implementation, and
  • the impact of programme implementation on the spread of HIV.

– In heavily affected countries, organizations have to cope with increased poverty among target groups and communities due to the chronic sickness and death of young and productive community members, increasing number of orphans, and increasing poverty and hunger. Rising poverty levels result in a lack of community resources and capacity to contribute to programmes and reduce programme sustainability.

> Mainstreaming HIV/AIDS addresses the impact of the epidemic on programme implementation and the impact of programme implementation on the spread of HIV.

– In countries and settings with lower HIV prevalence, HIV/AIDS is likely to impact on programme sustainability in the future if no adequate measures are taken.

– In the past, programmes specifically targeted at HIV/AIDS prevention and care have often been the main avenue through which AIDS interventions were carried out. These programmes can be beneficial through their potential to break the silence and taboos around AIDS. However, they also carry the risk of making AIDS a "special" issue, thereby hiding the fact that HIV/AIDS affects all aspects of people's lives.

- It may be necessary to provide additional activities to address HIV/AIDS alongside other interventions.
- Teaching and raising awareness of HIV/AIDS is a tool for mainstreaming HIV/AIDS in programme activities. The topic should be integrated into all curricula (e.g. agricultural/development projects, theological training, income-generating projects, etc.).
- Mainstreaming HIV/AIDS can be a tool for community empowerment: HIV/AIDS can be a subject in formal and informal discussions at community level; communities can be empowered to demand their rights; in agricultural programmes, promotion of farming techniques that take into consideration the loss of agricultural workers can help to mitigate the impact of HIV/AIDS; empowerment of women, particularly widows, to claim ownership of land, will reduce women's vulnerability to HIV; HIV testing and counselling can be promoted through programme activities.
- Organizations can embark on advocacy and lobbying at the local and national level on behalf of PLWHA and other vulnerable groups. This can relate to access to treatment and care, including antiretroviral treatment, human rights, etc. Churches in particular have the potential to play a decisive role and have a strong voice in advocacy.
- HIV/AIDS education should provide information on care options, particularly on ARV treatment. Such "treatment literacy" is of vital importance: increased access to ARV requires educating health workers, PLWHA and communities at large on all treatment related issues.
- *All* programmes can potentially increase the spread of HIV/AIDS. For example, projects that enhance migration can contribute to increasing HIV incidence; programme staff can contribute through their behaviour to increased transmission.
- To avoid programmes actually increasing the spread of HIV/AIDS, directly or indirectly, their impact on the transmission of HIV should be examined.

> To avoid programmes actually increasing the spread of HIV/AIDS, directly or indirectly, their impact on the transmission of HIV should be examined.

20. Literature

Abuja Declaration (2001). http://www.oau.org/afrsummit/docs.htm

Africa Comprehensive HIV/AIDS Partnership and Government of Botswana: Ntwa e Bolotse: Botswana's War Against AIDS. Satellite Meeting bei der 14. Internationalen AIDS Konferenz in Barcelona, 7–12 July 2002

Ahmed S et al. (2001). HIV incidence and sexually transmitted disease prevalence associated with condom use: a population study in Rakai, Uganda. *AIDS* 15: 2171–9

Asiimwe-Okiror G, Opio AA, Musinguzi J et al. (1997). Change in sexual behaviour and decline in HIV infection among young pregnant women in urban Uganda. *AIDS* 15: 11 (14), 1757–63

Attaran A and Gillespie-White L (2001). Do patents for antiretroviral drugs constrain access to AIDS treatment? *Journal of the American Medical Association* 286 (15): 1886–92

Attaran A and Sachs J (2001). Defining and redefining international donor support for combating the AIDS pandemic. *Lancet* 357 (9249): 57–61

Auvert B, Buvé A, Lagarde E et al. (2001). Male circumcision and HIV infection in four cities in sub-Saharan Africa. AIDS 15, Suppl 4: 31–40

Bartlett JA, DeMasia R, Quinn J et al. (2001). Overview of the effectiveness of triple combination therapy in antiretroviral-naive HIV-1 infected adults. *AIDS* 15: 1369–77

Benn C (2002a). The influence of cultural and religious frameworks on the future course of the HIV/AIDS epidemic. *Journal of Theology for Southern Africa* 113: 3–18

Benn C (2002b). HIV/AIDS. In Biesalski, HK; Köhrle J; Schümann K (eds): *Vitamine, Spurenelemente und Mineralstoffe*. Thieme Verlag, Stuttgart, 470–6

Benn C and Hyder A (2002). Equity and resource allocation in health care: dialogue between Islam and Christianity. *Medicine, Health Care and Philosophy* 5, 181–9

Botswana (2000). Human Development Report.

Brooks Jackson J, Musoke P, Fleming T et al. (2003). Intrapartum and neonatal single-dose nevirapine compared with zidovudine for prevention of mother-to-child transmission of HIV-1 in Kampala, Uganda: 18-month follow-up of the HIVNET 012 randomized trial. *Lancet* 362, Sept. 13: 859–68

Buvé A, Caraël M, Hayes RJ et al. (2001). The multicentre study on factors determining the differential spread of HIV in four African cities: summary and conclusions. *AIDS* 15 (suppl 4): 127–31

Byamugisha G (2000). *How can religious institutions talk about sexual matters?* Kampala, Uganda

Commission on Macroeconomics and Health (CMH) (2001). Investing in health for economic development. Report of the Commission on Macroeconomics and Health. WHO, Geneva. http://www3.who.int/whosis/menu.cfm?path=whosis,cmh&language=english

Consten ECJ, van Lanshot JB, Henry PC et al. (1995). A prospective study on the risk of exposure to HIV during surgery in Zambia. *AIDS* 9: 585–8

Coutsoudis A, Pillay K, Spooner E et al. (1999). Influence of infant-feeding patterns on early mother-to-child transmission of HIV-1 in Durban, South Africa: a prospective cohort study. *Lancet* 354: 471–6

Department of Health Government of South Africa (2003). Cabinet's decision on the operational plan for comprehensive care and treatment for people living with HIV and AIDS. http://www.doh.gov.za/docs/pr/pr1119-f.html

Ecumenical Advocacy Alliance (2001a). *HIV/AIDS Campaign*. http://www.e-alliance.ch/hivaids.htm

Ecumenical Advocacy Alliance (2001b). *Plan of Action*. http://www.e-alliance.ch/hivaidsplan.htm

Ecumenical Consultation on HIV/AIDS (2001). Plan of Action. http://www.wcc-coe.org/wcc/news/press/01/44pre.html

Editorial (2001a). China faces AIDS. *Lancet* 358 (9284)

Editorial (2001b). Patent protection versus public health. *Lancet* 358 (9293): 1563

Erskine S (2001). Current trends in HIV prevalence in Botswana, Namibia, South Africa and Swaziland. *AIDS Analysis Africa* Aug./Sept. 12 (2): 9–13

Esparza J (2001). Laying groundwork for AIDS vaccines in developing countries. IAVI Report – *The Newsletter on International AIDS Vaccine Research* 5 (7): 9–12

FAO (Food and Agricultural Organization) (2001). *Focus: AIDS – a threat to rural Africa*. http://www.fao.org/Focus/E/aids/aids6-e.htm

FAO (Food and Agricultural Organization) (2002). *AIDS hitting African farm sector hard*. http://www.fao.org/worldfoodsummit/english/newsroom/focus/focus4.htm

Farmer P, Léandre F, Mukherjee AS et al. (2001). Community-based approaches to HIV treatment in resource-poor settings. *Lancet* 358: 404–9

Fylkesnes K, Musonda RM, Sichone M et al. (2001). Declining HIV prevalence and risk behaviours in Zambia: evidence from surveillance and population-based surveys. *AIDS* 15 (7): 907–16

Gibson D, Flynn M, Perales D (2001). Effectiveness of syringe exchange programs in reducing HIV risk behavior and HIV seroconversion among injecting drug users. *AIDS* 15: 1329–41

Gisselquist D, Potterat JJ, Brody S, et al. (2003). Let it be sexual: how health care transmission of AIDS in Africa was ignored. *International Journal of STD and AIDS* 14 (3): 148–61

Global AIDS Surveillance (2001). *Weekly Epidemiological Record* 50, 14 Dec.

Global Fund to Fight AIDS, Malaria and Tuberculosis (2003). http://www.theglobalfund.org/en/

Global HIV Prevention Working Group (2002). *Global mobilization for HIV prevention.* http://www.gatesfoundation.org/nr/downloads/globalhealth/aids/hivprevreport_final.pdf

Goemaere E, Kaninda AV, Ciaffi L et al. (2002). Do patents prevent access to drugs for HIV in developing countries? *Journal of the American Medical Association* 287 (7): 841

Gray RH, Wawer MJ, Brookmeye R et al. and the Rakai Project Team (2001). Probability of HIV-1 transmission per coital act in monogamous, heterosexual, HIV-1 discordant couples in Rakai, Uganda. *Lancet* 357: 1149–53

Green EC (1999). *Indigenous theories of contagious disease.* AltaMira Press, Walnut Creek

Green EC (2003). Faith-based organizations: contributions to HIV prevention. USAID document, Synergy Project. http://www.usaid.gov/pop_health/aids/TechAreas/community/fbo.pdf

Gregson S, Nyamukapa CA, Garnett GP et al. (2002). Sexual mixing patterns and sex-differentials in teenage exposure to HIV infection in rural Zimbabwe. *Lancet* 359 (9321): 1896–903

Greyling C (2001). *HIV/AIDS and poverty – a challenge to the church in the new millennium.* Institute for theological and interdisciplinary research (EFSA), South Africa

Grosskurth H, Mosha F, Todd J et al. (1995). Impact of improved treatment of sexually transmitted diseases on HIV infection in rural Tanzania: randomized controlled trial. *Lancet* 346 (8974): 530–6

Grosskurth K, Gray R, Hayes R et al. (2000). Control of sexually transmitted diseases for HIV-1 prevention: understanding the implications of the Mwanza and Rakai trials. *Lancet* 355 (9219): 1981

Guay LA, Musoke P, Fleming T et al. (1999). Intrapartum and neonatal single-dose nevirapine compared with zidovudine for prevention of mother-to-child transmission of HIV-1 in Kampala, Uganda: HIVNET 012 randomized trial. *Lancet* 354: 795–802

Henderson DK et al. (1990). Risk for occupational transmission of HIV-1 associated with clinical exposure. *Annals of Internal Medicine* 113: 740–6

Human Sciences Research Council (2002). Nelson Mandela/HSRC study of HIV/AIDS. Household survey 2002. http://www.hsrc.ac.za

International Labour Organization (2001). *An ILO Code of Practice on HIV/AIDS and the world of work.* International Labour Office, Geneva http://www.ilo.org/public/english/protection/trav/download/hiv_a4_e.pdf

Individual members of the faculty of Harvard University (2001). Consensus statement on antiretroviral treatment for AIDS in poor countries.

http://www.cid.harvard.edu/cidinthenews/pr/consensus_aids_therapy.pdf

International Treatment Access Coalition (2002). http://www.itacoalition.org/

Kasper T, Hilderbrand K, Tshabane N et al. (2002). Antiretroviral therapy in primary health care centers in a South African township. *Abstract MoOrB1095*, presented at 14th International AIDS Conference, Barcelona, 7–12 July

Kelly MJ (2000). What HIV/AIDS can do to education in Zambia, and what education can do to HIV/AIDS. Presentation at 12th International Conference on AIDS and STDs in Africa (ICASA), Sept. 1999 http://www.sedos.org/english/kelly_1.htm

Kilmarx PH, Supawitkul S, Wankrairoj, M et al. (2000). Explosive spread and effective control of human immunodeficiency virus in northernmost Thailand: the epidemic in Chiang Mai Province, 1988–99. *AIDS* 14: 2731–40

Laga M, Schwartlander B, Pisani E et al. (2001). To stem HIV in Africa, prevent transmission to young women. *AIDS* 15: 931–4

Lagarde E, Auvert B, Caraël M et al. (2001). Condom use and its association with HIV/sexually transmitted diseases in four urban communities of sub-Saharan Africa. *AIDS* 15 (suppl 4): S71–8

Laurent C, Diakhaté N, Gueye NFN et al. (2002). The Senegalese government's highly active antiretroviral therapy initiative: an 18-month follow-up study. *AIDS* 16 (10): 1363–70

Magesa L (2000). Recognizing the reality of African religion in Tanzania. In JF Keenan (ed.) *Catholic Ethicists on HIV/AIDS Prevention*, Continuum, New York, 76–84

Malungo JR (2001). Sexual cleansing (Kusalazya) and levirate marriage (Kunjilila mung'anda) in the era of AIDS: changes in perceptions and practices in Zambia. *Social Science and Medicine* 53 (3): 371–82

Maman S, Mbwambo J, Hogan KM et al. (2001). Women's barriers to HIV-1 testing and disclosure: challenges for HIV-1 voluntary counselling and testing. *AIDS Care* 13 (5): 595–603

MAP Monitoring the AIDS Pandemic (2001). *The status and trends of HIV/AIDS/STI epidemics in Asia and the Pacific. Provisional report.* http://www.unaids.org/hivaidsinfo/statistics/MAP/index.html

Marseille E, Hoffmann PB, Kahn JG (2002). HIV prevention before HAART in sub-Saharan Africa. *Lancet* 359 (9320): 1851

McCarthy M (2003). AIDS vaccine fails in Thai trial. *Lancet* 362 (9397): 1728

Médecins sans Frontières (MSF) (2003b). Recent reports and publications. http://www.accessmed-msf.org/publications.shtm

Médecins sans Frontières, Consumer Project on Technology, Oxfam, Health Action International (2002). *Conference report: Implementation of the Doha Declaration on the TRIPS agreement and public health: how to get it right*. http://www.accessmed-msf.org/prod/publications.asp?scntid=22220021548172&contenttype=PARA&

Ministry of Health Tanzania/Gesellschaft für Technische Zusammenarbeit (2000). *Hope for Tanzania: lessons learned from a decade of comprehensive AIDS control in Mbeya region.* http://www.gtz.de/aids/download/heft_1.pdf

Moore A, Herrera G, Nyamongo J et al. (2001). Estimated risk of HIV transmission by blood transfusion in Kenya. *Lancet* 358 (9282): 657–60

Mwakagile D, Mmari E, Makwaya C et al. (2001). Sexual behaviour among youths at high risk for HIV-1 infection in Dar es Salaam, Tanzania. *Sexually Transmitted Infections* 77 (4): 255–9

National Intelligence Council (2002). The next wave of HIV/AIDS: Nigeria, Ethiopia, Russia, India and China (Sept.). http://www.cia.gov/nic/pubs/index.htm

Newell ML (1998). Mechanisms and timing of mother-to-child transmission of HIV-1. *AIDS* 12: 831–7

NIAID/NIH/DHHS (2001): *Workshop summary – scientific evidence on condom effectiveness for sexually transmitted disease (STD) prevention*, 20 July

Nieuwerk PT et al. (2001). Long-term quality of life outcomes in three antiretroviral treatment strategies for HIV-1 infection. *AIDS* 15: 1985–91

Nsutebu EF, Walley JD, Mataka E, Simon CF (2001). Scaling-up HIV/AIDS and TB home-based care: lessons from Zambia. *Health Policy and Planning* 16 (3): 240–7

Nyambedha EO, Wandibba S, Aagard-Hansen J (2001). Policy implications of the inadequate support systems for orphans in western Kenya. *Health Policy* 58 (1): 83–96

OHCHR/UNAIDS (2002). HIV/AIDS and human rights: Guideline 6. (Sept.) http://www.unaids.org/publications/documents/human/HIVAIDSHumanRights_Guideline6.pdf

Okware S, Opio A, Musinguzi J, Waibale P (2001). Fighting HIV/AIDS: is success possible? *Bulletin of the World Health Organization* 79 (12): 1113–19

Orrell C, Bangsberg DR, Badri M et al. (2003). Adherence is not a barrier to successful antiretroviral therapy in South Africa. *AIDS* 17 (9), 1369–76

Osborne CM (1996). Comprehensive care across a continuum. *AIDS* (10), Suppl 3: 61–7

Oxfam (2002). HIV/AIDS and food insecurity. Joint report from Oxfam and Save the Children

Palmore Beckermann K (2003). Long-term findings of HIVNET 012: the next steps. *Lancet* 362 (9387): 842–3

PANOS (2002). Patents, pills and public health – can TRIPS deliver? http://www.panos.org.uk/briefing/TRIPS_front.htm

Piot P, Coll-Seck A (2001). International response to the HIV/AIDS epidemic: planning for success. *Bulletin of the World Health Organization* 79 (12): 1106–12

Ruhl C, Pokrovsky V, Vinograd V (2002). The economic consequences of HIV in Russia. World Bank Group. http://www.worldbank.org.ru/eng/group/hiv/

Schwartlander B, Stover J, Walker N et al. (2001). Resource needs for HIV/AIDS. *Science* 29 June, 292 (5526): 2434–43

South Africa Department of Health (2002). *National HIV and syphilis sero-prevalence survey in South Africa*, 2001. http://196.36.153.56/doh/aids/index.html

South Africa Department of Health (2003). Cabinet decision on Care and Treatment for People living with HIV and AIDS. http://www.doh.gov.za/aids/index.html

South African Medical Research Council (2001). *The impact of HIV/AIDS on adult mortality in South Africa*. http://www.mrc.ac.ta/bod

South Asia Ecumenical Partnership Programme (SAEPP) (2003). Guidelines. http://www.wcc-coe.org/wcc/what/regional/saepp-guidelines.pdf

Stoneburner R (2000). Analyses of HIV trend and behavioral data in Uganda, Kenya, and Zambia: prevalence declines in Uganda relate more to reduction in sex partners than condom use. *Abstract ThOrC72*, presented at 13th International AIDS Conference, Durban

Stover J, Walker N, Garnett GP et al. (2002). Can we reverse the HIV/AIDS pandemic with an expanded response? *Lancet* 360 (9326): 73–7

Sweat M, Gregorich S, Sangiwa G et al. (2000). Cost-effectiveness of voluntary HIV-1 counselling and testing in reducing sexual transmission of HIV-1 in Kenya and Tanzania. *Lancet* 356 (9224): 113–21

Tarantola D (2001). Facing the reality of AIDS – a 15-year process? *Bulletin of the World Health Organization* 79 (12): 1095

TASO (The AIDS Support Organization) (2000). Living positively with AIDS. http://www.taso.co.ug/

The Voluntary HIV-1 counselling and testing Efficacy Group (2000). Efficacy of voluntary HIV-1 counselling and testing in individuals and couples in Kenya, Tanzania, and Trinidad: a randomized trial. *Lancet* 356: 103–12

Treatment Action Campaign. 2003. http://www.tac.org.za/

UNAIDS (1997). Impact of HIV and sexual health education on the sexual behaviour of young people: a review update. UNAIDS, Geneva

UNAIDS (1999). *Peer education and HIV/AIDS: Concepts, uses and challenges*. UNAIDS, Geneva

UNAIDS (1999a). Gender and HIV/AIDS: Taking stock of research and pogrammes. UNAIDS, Geneva

UNAIDS (2000a). *Opening up the HIV/AIDS epidemic. Guidance on encouraging beneficial disclosure, ethical partner counselling and appropriate use of HIV case reporting.* http://www.unaids.org/publications/documents/hivnotification/files/JC-ExecSumm-E.pdf

UNAIDS (2000b). *Global strategy framework on HIV/AIDS. UNAIDS*, Geneva

UNAIDS (2001a). *AIDS epidemic update* – December 2001 http://www.unaids.org/epidemic_update/report_dec01/index.html#full

UNAIDS (2001b). *Uganda: HIV and AIDS-related discrimination, stigmatization and denial.* http://www.unaids.org/publications/documents/care/general/JC590-Uganda-E.pdf

UNAIDS (2001c). *Population mobility and AIDS.* UNAIDS, Geneva

UNAIDS (2001d). HIV/AIDS: Global crisis – Global action. United Nations Special Session on HIV/AIDS Fact Sheets. http://www.unaids.org/fact_sheets/ungass/index.html

UNAIDS (2001e). HIV causing tuberculosis cases to double in Africa. www.unaids.org/whatsnew/press/eng/pressarc01/TB_240401.html

UNAIDS (2002). Report on the global HIV/AIDS epidemic. http://www.unaids.org/barcelona/presskit/report.html

UNAIDS (2003). AIDS epidemic update. December. http://www.unaids.org/en/default.asp

UNAIDS/UNICEF (2002). Children on the brink: A joint report on orphan estimates and program strategies. http://www.unaids.org/barcelona/presskit/childrenonthebrink.html

UNAIDS/WHO (2001). *Fighting HIV-related intolerance: exposing the links between racism, stigma and discrimination.* http://www.unaids.org/humanrights/BPracism.doc

UNFPA (2002). State of the world's population: people, poverty and possibilities. http://www.unfpa.org/swp/swpmain.htm

UNHCR (United Nations High Commissioner for Refugees) (2001). *Refugees and HIV.* http://www.unhcr.ch/cgi-bin/texis/vtx/home/+EwwBmWeDEudwwwwwwwwwwwhFqh0kgZTtFqnnLnqAFqh0kgZTcFqmroVDzmxwwwwww/opendoc.pdf

UNICEF(n.d.). My future is my choice – Life skills programme Namibia. http://www.unicef.org/programme/hiv/focus/youth/nama.htm

UNICEF (2000a). *State of the world's children 2001.* UNICEF, New York

UNICEF (2000b). *Progress of nations 2000.* UNICEF, New York. http://www.unicef.org/pubsgen/pon00/index.html

UNICEF (2001a). State of the world's children 2002. UNICEF, New York

UNICEF (2001b) UNICEF warns: Demand for child sex is linked to spread of HIV/AIDS. UNICEF *Press release*, 28 Nov. http://www.unicef.org/newsline/01pr93.htm

UNICEF/UNAIDS/WHO (2002). *Young people and HIV/AIDS: opportunity in crisis.* http://www.unicef.org/pubsgen/youngpeople-hivaids/youngpeople-hivaids.pdf

UNICEF/WHO/UNAIDS (1998a). *HIV and infant feeding: a review of HIV transmission through breastfeeding.*

United Nations (1966a). *International Covenant on Economic, Social and Cultural Rights.* http://www.unhchr.ch/html/menu3/b/a_cescr.htm

United Nations (1966b). *International Covenant on Civil and Political Rights.* http://www.unhchr.ch/html/menu3/b/a_cescr.htm

United Nations (2001). *General Assembly Special Session on HIV/AIDS Declaration of Commitment.* http://www.unaids.org/UNGASS/index.html

United Nations Office for Drug Control and Crime Prevention, Regional Office for Russia and Belarus (2002). *Country Profile Russian Federation*, Moscow

Urassa M, Boerma JT, Isingo R et al. (2001). The impact of HIV/AIDS on mortality and household mobility in rural Tanzania. *AIDS* 15 (15): 2017–23

Van Damme L, Ramjee G, Alary M et al. (2002). Effectiveness of COL-1492, a nonoxynol-9 vaginal gel, on HIV-1 transmission in female sex workers: a randomized controlled trial. *Lancet* 360: 971–7

Wawer MJ, Sewankambo NK, Serwadda D et al. (1999). Control of sexually transmitted diseases for AIDS prevention in Uganda: a randomized community trial. Rakai Project Study Group. *Lancet* 353 (9152): 525–35

Weidle PJ, Malamba S, Mwebaze R et al. (2002). Assessment of a pilot antiretroviral drug therapy programme in Uganda: patients' response, survival and drug resistance. *Lancet* 360: 34–40

Weinreich S (2002). Menschenrechte und internationale Zusammenarbeit am Beispiel des Zugangs zu antiretroviralen Medikamenten für die Aids-Behandlung. In *Social Watch Report Deutschland*, Nr.2, hrsg. vom Deutschen NRO-Forum Weltsozialgipfel

Wendo C (2001). Most Ugandan HIV-positive mothers insist on breast-feeding. *Lancet* 359 (9282)

WHO (2000). DOTS. http://www.who.int/gtb/dots/index.htm

WHO (2001) Technical Consultation. *New data on the prevention of mother-to-child transmission of HIV and their policy implications: conclusions and recommendations.* http://www.unaids.org/publications/documents/mtct/MTCT_Consultation_Report.doc

WHO (2002a). Scaling up antiretroviral therapy in resource-limited settings: Guidelines for a public health approach. http://www.who.int/hiv/pub/prev_care/draft/en/

WHO (2002b). Access to HIV drugs and diagnostics of acceptable quality. http://www.who.int/medicines/organization/qsm/activities/pilotproc/suppliers.doc

WHO (2002c). Essential drugs and medicines policy: 12th Expert Committee on the selection and use of essential medicines, 12–19 April. http://www.who.int/medicines/organization/par/edl/expert-comm.shtml

WHO/UNAIDS (1998). *Policy statement on preventive therapy against tuberculosis in people living with HIV*. WHO, Geneva

WHO/UNAIDS (2000). Key elements in HIV/AIDS care and support. http://www.who.int/HIV_AIDS/HIV_AIDS_Care/Key_elements_HIV_AIDS_care.htm

WHO/FRH/NUT/CHD/98.3, UNAIDS/98.5, UNICEF/PD/NUT/(J)98-3 UNICEF/WHO/UNAIDS (1998b). *HIV and infant feeding: a guide for health care managers and supervisors.*

WHO/FRH/NUT/CHD/98.2, UNAIDS/98.4, UNICEF/PD/NUT/(J)98-2 United Nations Commission on Human Rights (2001). Access to medication in the context of pandemics such as HIV/AIDS. http://www.unhchr.ch/huridocda/huridoca.nsf/(symbol)/E.CN.4.RES.2001.33.En?Opendocu

World Bank (1997) *Confronting AIDS: Public Health Priorities in a Global Epidemic.* Oxford University Press, New York

World Council of Churches (1987). Minutes of the 38th meeting of the WCC central committee. WCC, Geneva

World Council of Churches (1997). Facing AIDS – the challenge, the churches' response. *WCC Study Document*, WCC Publications, Geneva

World Council of Churches (2001). Statement by faith-based organizations facilitated by the World Council of Churches for the UN Special General Assembly on HIV/AIDS. *International Review of Mission* 90 (359): 473–6

WTO (1994). *Agreement on trade-related aspects of intellectual property rights.* WTO, New York. http://www.wto.org/english/tratop_e/trips_e/implem_para6_e.htm

WTO (2001). Declaration on the TRIPS agreement and public health. Adopted 14 Nov. http://www.wto.org/english/thewto_e/minist_e/min01_e/mindecl_trips_e.htm

WTO (2003). Implementation of paragraph 6 of the Doha Declaration on the TRIPS Agreement and public health. Decision of the General Council of 30 August.

Yamba, Bawa C (1997) Cosmologies in turmoil: witchfinding and AIDS in Chiawa, Zambia. *Africa* 67: 216–23